T0099955

Developing Public Health Interventions

Sara Miller McCune founded SAGE Publishing in 1965 to support the dissemination of usable knowledge and educate a global community. SAGE publishes more than 1000 journals and over 800 new books each year, spanning a wide range of subject areas. Our growing selection of library products includes archives, data, case studies and video. SAGE remains majority owned by our founder and after her lifetime will become owned by a charitable trust that secures the company's continued independence.

Los Angeles | London | New Delhi | Singapore | Washington DC | Melbourne

Developing Public Health Interventions

A Step-by-Step Guide

Ruth Jepson
John McAteer
Andrew James Williams
Larry Doi
Audrey Buelo

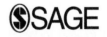

Los Angeles | London | New Delhi
Singapore | Washington DC | Melbourne

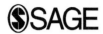

Los Angeles | London | New Delhi
Singapore | Washington DC | Melbourne

SAGE Publications Ltd
1 Oliver's Yard
55 City Road
London EC1Y 1SP

SAGE Publications Inc.
2455 Teller Road
Thousand Oaks, California 91320

SAGE Publications India Pvt Ltd
B 1/I 1 Mohan Cooperative Industrial Area
Mathura Road
New Delhi 110 044

SAGE Publications Asia-Pacific Pte Ltd
3 Church Street
#10-04 Samsung Hub
Singapore 049483

© Ruth Jepson John McAteer 2022
First published 2022

Editor: Alex Clabburn
Assistant editor: Ruth Lilly
Production editor: Sarah Cooke
Copyeditor: Jane Robson
Proofreader: Sharon Cawood
Indexer: Melanie Gee
Marketing manager: George Kimble
Cover design: Sheila Tong
Typeset by: C&M Digitals (P) Ltd, Chennai, India
Printed in the UK

Library of Congress Control Number: 2021940988

British Library Cataloguing in Publication data

A catalogue record for this book is available from the British Library

ISBN 978-1-5297-3242-9
ISBN 978-1-5297-3241-2 (pbk)

At SAGE we take sustainability seriously. Most of our products are printed in the UK using FSC papers and boards. When we print overseas we ensure sustainable papers are used as measured by the PREPS grading system. We undertake an annual audit to monitor our sustainability.

This book is dedicated to anyone working with individuals and communities to create sustainable, positive change and those learning how to do so. This book and the tools within it are for you.

CONTENTS

Acknowledgements   ix

About the Authors   x

1   Introduction to the book   1
   Ruth Jepson

2   Principles of intervention development   13
   Ruth Jepson and John McAteer

3   Causality, systems and complexity   36
   Ruth Jepson, Andrew J. Williams and Lawrence Doi

4   6SQuID Step 1: Understanding the problem and its causes   59
   Ruth Jepson, Lawrence Doi and Audrey Buelo

5   6SQuID Step 2: Identifying modifiable causal factors   80
   Ruth Jepson and John McAteer

**6   6SQuID Step 3: Identifying how to bring about change:
     theory of change**   104
   John McAteer and Ruth Jepson

**7   6SQuID Step 4: Identifying how to deliver change
     mechanisms – theory of action**   134
   John McAteer and Ruth Jepson

8   6SQuID Step 5: Testing and adapting the intervention   157
   John McAteer, Lawrence Doi, Audrey Buelo and Ruth Jepson

**9   6SQuID Step 6: Collecting sufficient evidence of effectiveness
     to proceed to a rigorous evaluation**   174
   Andrew J. Williams

10 Case studies   194
   Ruth Jepson and John McAteer
   Case study 1. HIV infection and treatment adherence   195
   *Caroline Masquillier, Edwin Wouters, Linda Campbell, Anton Delport,
   Neo Sematlane, Lorraine Tanyaradzwa Dube and Lucia Knight*

Case study 2. Sedentary behaviour in contact centres   201
Divya Sivaramakrishnan and Ruth Jepson
Case study 3. Physical activity in women at high risk of type 2 diabetes   210
Audrey Buelo
Case study 4. ManaiaSAFE Forestry School   216
Marg Wilkie and Henry Koia

11 Conclusion   **223**
John McAteer and Ruth Jepson

Glossary   234
Index   238

ACKNOWLEDGEMENTS

We would like to thank Professor Daniel Wight and Dr Erica Wimbush who contributed to the original development of the 6SQuID framework. We would also like to thank Dr Divya Sivaramakrishnan, Dr Caroline Masquillier, Henry Koia and Dr Marg Wilkie for kindly writing case studies for inclusion in this book, in addition to Christine Roseveare and Shauni Burke. Over the past six years, our thinking on the 6SQuID framework has developed into the material within this book. We would like to thank all of those we have worked with, including both our non-academic and academic colleagues and the students who attended our course on the MPH at the University of Edinburgh.

ABOUT THE AUTHORS

Professor Ruth Jepson is a professor of public health in social science and Director of the Scottish Collaboration for Public Health Research and Policy at the University of Edinburgh. She has a background in nursing and has worked in the field of public health for over 30 years. Her expertise includes systematic reviews, co-production, qualitative methods and the development and evaluation of complex public health interventions. She was part of the team which developed the Six Steps in Quality Intervention Development and has used it widely in her teaching and research.

Dr John McAteer MSc PhD is a chartered psychologist and Associate Fellow of the British Psychological Society. John's expertise is in behaviour change, public health and the development and evaluation of complex interventions. Over the past 18 years, John has led and been involved with many intervention projects, working closely with policy makers and practitioners. His work has fed into national policy initiatives such as the Scottish Government's National Parenting Strategy. He is currently a co-director of Grow Public Health Research and Consultancy, in Edinburgh, UK.

Dr Andrew James Williams MPH PhD FHEA is a senior lecturer in Public Health at the University of St Andrews, UK. Andrew has been involved with the evaluation of nation-wide (abolition of prescription fees) and city-wide policies (20mph speed limits) through to smaller-scale youth work and community development interventions. Having trained in quantitative methods (epidemiology), Andrew's interests are now in what sustains and improves our health, which means grappling with the complex systems that influence health. He is particularly keen that we learn from all interventions through thorough evaluation.

Dr Lawrence Doi BSc MPH PhD FHEA is a lecturer in Applied Public Health and Postgraduate Research Director (Nursing Studies) at the University of Edinburgh, UK. His expertise is in developing and evaluating complex interventions. Lawrence taught on the developing and evaluating complex intervention course at masters level for five years. He has been involved in several intervention development projects, including leading a team of researchers and stakeholders to develop an intervention to reduce high readmission rates for patients following intensive care admission. He is currently the lead researcher on a Scottish Government-funded project evaluating the universal health visiting pathway.

Dr Audrey Buelo MPH PhD is an epidemiologist studying the COVID-19 vaccination response at Public Health Scotland. She received her Doctorate in Applied Health and Social Sciences at the University of Edinburgh. Her doctoral research involved the development of a physical activity and mental health improvement intervention for women who are at high risk of type 2 diabetes through novel methods of co-production.

1

INTRODUCTION TO THE BOOK

This textbook provides a practical guide to the stages of intervention development. It will assist practitioners and researchers in the development of effective, acceptable and sustainable interventions. These could be policies, programmes or services. Current intervention development tools and frameworks tend to be complex, highly technical and not well suited to intervention development in the real world. The book utilises the **Six Steps in Quality Intervention Development (6SQuID)** framework to provide a pragmatic method of creating effective and sustainable interventions for a wide variety of populations and settings. It not only provides you with an understanding of the theory and concepts behind intervention development, but also a range of tools you can use to develop a sustainable and effective intervention.

This textbook focuses on social interventions to improve public health, including the social aspects of interventions with clinical outcomes, such as immunisation programmes. However, the approach we use is relevant and useful for broader intervention development in other fields, including education, social interventions, psychology, criminal justice, environment and global health and development. This introductory chapter will describe the background and rationale for the Six Steps in Quality Intervention Development (6SQuID) framework, as well as other intervention development frameworks, and their strengths and weaknesses. The overall aim is to demonstrate the importance of developing interventions and using 6SQuID as an intervention development framework. This chapter will also introduce how the remaining chapters are structured.

Learning objectives

By the end of this chapter, you will understand:

- What an intervention is
- The importance of focusing on intervention development as much as intervention evaluation
- The basics of 6SQuID
- What 6SQuID adds to the existing methods of developing interventions
- Who should use 6SQuID and why.

WHAT IS AN INTERVENTION?

For the purposes of this book, we are defining an **intervention** as a *planned action* (or set of actions) that is designed to bring about a *desired change* (of one or more outcomes) in a defined population to address a social or health problem. Interventions may be called programmes, policies, services or projects, but their common aim is to 'intervene' to have a desired effect. Examples include:

- A smoking ban (planned action) in the general population within a country (defined population) to reduce lung diseases (outcome) caused by cigarette smoking (health problem)
- A peer support group (planned action) in schools (defined population) to reduce alcohol use (outcome) caused by social norms and peer pressure (problem).

Interventions are often developed or implemented in response to a 'problem' (e.g. high levels of smoking, an outbreak of cholera) when there are either no interventions in place or none which are creating the desired effect. In public health, education or social services, the desired changes are usually around improving health, educational or societal outcomes.

The range of interventions is endless, and humans have always sought to intervene to make their lives and those of their families and communities more secure, healthier and better. So whilst interventions have been around for centuries, and many are very effective, we are still faced with a world where there are health conditions which seem to resist many interventions in place (e.g. diabetes, depression), new ones appearing (e.g. COVID-19) and potentially new threats to come. To be responsive and effective, we must understand how and why interventions work.

Some of you may have already started to ask questions such as 'What happens if there is more than one cause?' For example, in the case of alcohol use in young people, the causes could include the availability of alcohol or cultural norms. We know that outcomes such as obesity or poor educational attainment are the result of a multitude of causes, which may vary from country to country. These and many other questions are answered in subsequent chapters. In this book, we will be focusing primarily on complex interventions, as those are the most common in public health and have application to the health-related social science disciplines. Intervention development to help us manage and understand complexity requires different approaches and ways of thinking. The methods used to develop such interventions are also much less well developed than in the medical or certain public health fields (e.g. vaccination) where development and evaluation of interventions are more straightforward.

Knowledge link: This topic is also covered in Chapter 3

We have written this book for students and practitioners who would like to understand and gain skills in the development of interventions, programmes, projects or policies which are aimed at changing some aspect of the social world. By social world, we mean the world outside the internal systems of the human body, particularly groups of individuals or populations. Taking a step-by-step approach, this book provides a pragmatic and effective method of developing and evaluating interventions in a variety of fields. It presents the 6SQuID framework in a manner that is ideally suited to a semester course. Relevant case studies have been carefully selected to further illustrate the practical application of the various steps of the framework.

WHY IS ROBUST INTERVENTION DEVELOPMENT IMPORTANT?

Scientific interest and approaches to the development of interventions started primarily in the medical field with the development of drug and surgical interventions. The development of drugs is underpinned by a thorough understanding of the biological and pathological causal pathways; much time is spent in laboratories, undertaking basic research to understand the underlying mechanisms or causes of a certain disease. For example, it is important to know about the pathogenesis of an infectious disease to develop an effective intervention to tackle it. It is now standard practice to develop drugs based on plausible causal pathways and is considered highly unethical to administer a drug without proper development and evaluation phases. Such work includes testing for safety, efficacy, tolerance and acceptability. Much time, money and effort are put into the development of new compounds and drugs. Once they are developed, their administration and implementation are usually relatively standardised, and there are rigorous protocols and guidelines for drug development and evaluation.

When we move beyond the world of drug and medical device development, into the world of more social interventions (e.g. services to reduce loneliness), we find that those who develop the interventions often do not fully consider the underlying causes, the mechanisms of action and the causal pathways. They often rely on 'intuition', expert knowledge and research from other areas. Whilst this method of developing interventions may result in some success (if any), much time and effort may also be spent on interventions that are not effective. Indeed, Leviton et al. (2010) state that many evaluations arrive at no-effect conclusions because 'the program in question was not fully developed, was fatally flawed, or was so *puny* in terms of the treatments actually being provided that a change in outcome could never hope to be achieved' (p. 215).

In the last few decades, the focus, effort and funding of intervention research in public health and related disciplines has been primarily spent on evaluation. The randomised controlled trial (RCT) and, more recently, natural experiment and realist evaluation methodologies are seen as being the primary way of demonstrating effectiveness and examining how interventions work. These methodological designs have been the cornerstone of evidence for developing new services and programmes. Evaluation methods have been very well developed and many papers written on how to conduct these. However, many of these methods make assumptions that may not necessarily be true. These assumptions include:

1. The intervention being evaluated (whether a school-based peer support programme or a speed reduction programme) is the *best* it can be.
2. The intervention will result in the anticipated changes (in outcomes).
3. There is a clear pathway from the intervention to the outcomes of interest.
4. The intervention can be implemented in real life without any loss of effectiveness.

The outputs of an RCT are often considered to be the gold standard since this design is thought to greatly reduce the likelihood of research bias, such as how participants are allocated to the intervention or control group. The RCT was developed primarily to evaluate the effects of drug trials and can do that very well. But there are several problems when we try to evaluate complex health interventions using RCTs. First, populations (of school children, offenders, smokers) do not behave in the same consistent ways that biological systems do. Second, the intervention often interacts with systems such as school and workplaces and the RCT is not designed to evaluate the impact of the interaction. Third, and more importantly for this book, they are often evaluating poorly conceptualised social interventions which have not considered the complexity of the world in which we live. In many countries, we can see this because although we spend millions on programmes and policies, the rates and magnitude of change of outcomes such as literacy, recidivism and obesity remain remarkably unchanged. Whilst this is not only because of poorly developed interventions, it undoubtedly contributes.

WHY USE THE SIX STEPS IN QUALITY INTERVENTION DEVELOPMENT (6SQuID)?

Improving the effectiveness of public health interventions relies as much on attention paid to their design and feasibility as that paid to evaluation. Yet, compared to the vast literature on how to evaluate interventions, there are only a few frameworks to guide researchers or practitioners on how best to develop such interventions in logical, evidence-based ways to maximise effectiveness.

A brief overview of the background to 6SQuID and its development

In 2014, a group of researchers in public health (Ruth Jepson, Daniel Wight, Erica Wimbush and Lawrence Doi) met to discuss the discrepancy between the large amount of effort, focus and funding spent on an evaluation of interventions compared with the development of interventions. This led to us writing a paper outlining 6SQuID (Wight et al., 2016) and in the intervening years we have further refined it through our teaching and research. The purpose of developing 6SQuID was to create a robust, practical framework for developing more theoretical, thoughtful, acceptable, effective and sustainable interventions in the social sciences. We also wanted it to be used in teaching. For several years, we taught it as a ten-week module called the 'Development and Evaluation of Complex Public Health Interventions' as part of a Masters of Public Health. Our teaching focused both on knowledge and skill building. As part of the course assessment, we asked teams of students to develop an intervention. One of the interventions that was developed during the second year of running the course went on to get significant UK funding, and we have just finished a pilot and feasibility study in relation to this. The intervention was called Stand Up for Health and we use it both as an example and as a case study in the book.

Other frameworks exist, such as Intervention Mapping (Bartholemew et al., 2006), the UK MRC guidance (Craig et al., 2013; O'Cathain et al., 2019) and PRECEDE-PROCEED (Green and Kreuter, 2005). These have all been widely used, but have some limitations as discussed below. The Intervention Mapping framework is one of the most widely used intervention development frameworks today. It is well regarded and provides a rigorous approach to intervention development using an elaborate framework. Whilst this provides a thorough description of how to develop a health promotion intervention, it is highly technical, lengthy and prescriptive – it can take years to develop and implement an intervention fully and it is difficult to operationalise. It is also limited to the health promotion field, whereas 6SQuID is generalisable to several different fields. It also does not take good account of systems.

The MRC Guidance for the Development and Evaluation of Complex Interventions identifies three broad stages of intervention development: developing theory, modelling process and outcomes, and assessing feasibility. However, this guidance does not break down these stages much further and focuses primarily on the evaluation stages rather than intervention development itself. New guidance based on the MRC guidance has been developed, but it is published only as an academic paper and as such is limited in terms of detail provided (O'Cathain et al., 2019).

The PRECEDE-PROCEED model is another intervention development and evaluation model primarily driven by the socio-ecological approach. The planning phase is PRECEDE; the evaluation is PROCEED. It is extensively data-driven and practical application requires great technical skill, time and money. It also does not provide specific details of intervention development.

This textbook aims to provide clear and concise information that addresses these issues, such as the lack of practical detail and hard-to-operationalise technical guidance. In essence, 6SQuID aims to hit an optimal middle ground between the 'too little' and the 'too much' information offered by existing frameworks. We aim to help the reader to develop the necessary skills to feel confident in developing an intervention from scratch. The steps, which will be discussed in depth in the following chapters, are summarised in Table 1.1.

Although these steps are numbered from one to six, suggesting a linear progression, in reality intervention development is dynamic and iterative to create something effective and sustainable. You will quickly discover that you need to move backwards and forwards between steps as you progress through your intervention development journey.

Table 1.1   The Six Steps in Quality Intervention Development

Step		Questions to be addressed
Step 1	Define and understand the problem and its causes	Is it well understood? Does everybody view it in the same way?
Step 2	Clarify which causal or contextual factors are malleable and have greatest scope for change	What is causing the problem? Are they individual, structural or organisational factors?
Step 3	Identify how to bring about change: the change mechanism	What do we know about how to bring about the change in outcomes?
Step 4	Identify how to deliver the change mechanism	What activities do we need to do to bring about the change?
Step 5	Test and refine on a small scale	What happens when we test it? Does it work as intended?
Step 6	Collect sufficient evidence of effectiveness to justify rigorous evaluation/implementation	Can we collect data on effectiveness? How do we link it into evaluation?

OVERVIEW OF THE BOOK

The book is primarily structured specifically around the 6SQuID steps. However, there are several considerations in intervention development which you should keep in mind when following these steps to ensure that your intervention is as good as it can be. These considerations include co-production, inequalities, ethics and sustainability. You will also need to understand complexity and systems.

Whilst the book may make intervention development look complex, it really does not have to be. Much of it you may already be doing unconsciously when you are devising activities and strategies in your personal or work life. What we are aiming to do is to encourage you to make more conscious decisions so that you can replicate your interventions if they turn out to be successful.

Chapter 2: Principles of intervention development

This chapter will introduce nine key principles in intervention development. Some of these may already be second nature to you; others may help you think differently about your approach. These are ideas and principles that should be considered throughout the intervention development process. These include: identifying the need for an intervention; co-production of interventions and engaging with partners; health and social inequalities; ethics in intervention development; identifying assets and using resources efficiently; and sustainability of interventions.

Chapter 3: Causality, complexity and systems

Throughout the book, we often talk about causality, complexity and systems, so this chapter will introduce these concepts. The chapter covers: what complexity means in terms of complex interventions; understanding differences in the definitions of interventions – simple, complex and complicated; understanding which systems interventions operate in; and understanding why complexity and systems are important for intervention development and evaluation.

Chapter 4: 6SQuID Step 1 – Understanding the problem and its causes

The first step of developing an intervention is to understand the problems and its causes. Step 1 creates the foundation for a successful intervention. This chapter will describe how to fully understand the problem an intervention is trying to address, including clarifying it with key stakeholders and decision makers, and how to identify the relevant data to understand the contributing factors to the problem.

Chapter 5: 6SQuID Step 2 – Identifying modifiable causal factors

Step 1, as described above, aims to help you identify and summarise the factors that are related to your problem. Amongst the contributory factors that shape a problem, some are likely to be more modifiable than others (for example, we may be able to modify or change travel routes, but we cannot modify the weather). The next step (Step 2) is to identify which have the greatest scope for change. This might be at any point along the causal chain. This chapter will describe the practical considerations that need to be accounted for when determining which factors to address in a future intervention, such as resource availability and timescales.

Chapter 6: 6SQuID Step 3 – Identifying how to bring about change: theory of change

Having identified the most promising modifiable causal or contextual factors to address, it is necessary to think through how to achieve that change. At the heart of all social interventions is an implicit or explicit *theory of change* about how the intervention is intended to bring about the desired changes or outcomes. This is also referred to as the 'change mechanism'. The theory of change is about the central processes or drivers by which change comes about for individuals, groups or communities, and how the intervention activates the change process. This chapter will explore how to create a theory of change, including how to demonstrate this visually using logic models. Short case studies and examples will illustrate how a theory of change is developed.

Chapter 7: 6SQuID Step 4 – Identifying how to deliver change mechanisms

This chapter will describe how to implement the theory of change that has been developed in the previous chapter, termed developing a *theory of action*. A theory of action is concerned with developing all the components (activities) of an intervention which will bring about the change. Sometimes a change can only be brought about through a very limited range of activities, for instance legal change is achieved through legislation. However, other changes can be activated in several ways. This chapter will also discuss what to consider when designing the intervention (e.g. who is most suited to deliver it and any training requirements), as well as potential obstacles (time, resources) and unintended outcomes, and how to address or mitigate these.

Chapter 8: 6SQuID Step 5 – Testing and adapting the intervention

The testing stage involves testing and refining your theory of change and theory of action so that it can be adapted and improved before full implementation. This step varies considerably according to the type of intervention and frequently this is the stage of intervention development that is most hurried, due to lack of resources and time. This chapter will emphasise the importance of careful, small-scale testing and refinement. It will also describe common problems and pitfalls when testing an intervention, with practical solutions for each.

Chapter 9: 6SQuID Step 6 – Collecting sufficient evidence of effectiveness to proceed to a rigorous evaluation

Once the intervention has been piloted and revised and is considered 'good enough' for full implementation, the final step in intervention development is to establish sufficient evidence of effectiveness to warrant proceeding. This could mean moving to a large-scale rigorous outcomes evaluation (which could be a randomised controlled trial, realist evaluation, stepped-wedge or natural experiment) or, if resources and time are constricted, as in many third-sector organisations, moving to wide-scale implementation. This chapter will describe how to evaluate an intervention to assess its effectiveness in a time- and cost-efficient manner, with an emphasis on the economics of scaling up an intervention.

Chapter 10: Case studies

This chapter will provide several real-world and international case studies of interventions that have successfully used the full six steps covered by the book, from defining the problem and understanding its causes to collecting sufficient evidence of effectiveness. This will allow the reader to understand how the framework can be applied in the real world. While the steps appear discrete, in reality there can be a fair amount of overlap between them – for example, understanding the factors that influence the problem can often be combined with clarifying modifiable factors. The case studies will provide a more advanced description of how 6SQuID can be used for different purposes – from a PhD study to a community project.

Chapter 11: Conclusion

The final chapter will provide a broad summary of 6SQuID, will contextualise it in today's world and give further detail on how it can be used in teaching. It will also describe the next steps of intervention implementation, transferability and sustainability, and provide suggestions for further reading on these topics.

> ## Activity 1.1
>
> ### Reflective Practice
>
> Think of an intervention (programme, policy or project) that you may have been involved in, or you have been affected by. It could be anything from a stop smoking campaign to a service to reduce unemployment amongst young people. Try and identify the problem it is addressing; the planned action(s); the change it was intended to make (e.g. the outcomes); and the population it was targeting. Ask yourself if you think that the intervention was well developed and able to create the anticipated change (e.g. getting people back into work, reducing smoking, increasing adherence to a vaccination).

CHAPTER SUMMARY

There has been less emphasis on intervention development than evaluation in the social sciences. This has resulted in many interventions being either ineffective or not reaching their full potential. A more systematic and transparent approach will lead to more effective, sustainable and acceptable interventions and make better use of scarce resources. The Six Steps in Quality Intervention Development (6SQuID) offers a framework which is easy to follow, based on robust research and demonstrated in a range of case studies. It has been designed to be applicable to different disciplines and geographical areas.

FURTHER READING

O'Cathain, A., Croot, L., Duncan, E., Rousseau, N., Sworn, K., Turner, K. M., et al. (2019) 'Guidance on how to develop complex interventions to improve health and health-care', *BMJ Open*, 9 (8): e029954.

Wight, D., Wimbush, E., Jepson, R., and Doi, L. (2016) 'Six steps in quality intervention development (6SQuID)', *Journal of Epidemiology and Community Health*, 70 (5): 520–5. doi: 10.1136/jech-2015-205952. Epub 16 November 2015. PMID: 26573236; PMCID: PMC4853546.

REFERENCES

Bartholomew, L. K., Parcel, G. S., Kok, G., and Gottlieb, N. H. (2006) *Planning Health Promotion Programs: An Intervention Mapping Approach*, 2nd ed., ed. H. Schaalma, C. Markham, S. Tyrrell, R. Shegog, M. Fernndez, P. D. Mullen, et al. San Francisco: Jossey-Bass.

Craig, P., Dieppe, P., Macintyre, S., Michie, S., Nazareth, I., and Petticrew, M. (2013) 'Developing and evaluating complex interventions: the new Medical Research Council guidance', *International Journal of Nursing Studies, 50* (5): 587–92.

Green, L. W., and Kreuter, M. W. (2005) *Health Program Planning: An Educational and Ecological Approach*, 4th edition. New York: McGraw-Hill.

Leviton, L. C., Khan, L. K., Rog, D., Dawkins, N., and Cotton, D. (2010) 'Evaluability assessment to improve public health policies, programs, and practices', *Annual Review of Public Health, 31*: 213–33.

O'Cathain, A., Croot, L., Duncan, E., Rousseau, N., Sworn, K., Turner, K. M., et al. (2019) 'Guidance on how to develop complex interventions to improve health and health-care', *BMJ open, 9*(8): e029954.

Wight, D., Wimbush, E., Jepson, R., and Doi, L. (2016) 'Six steps in quality intervention development (6SQuID)', *Journal of Epidemiology and Community Health, 70* (5): 520–5.

ACTIVITY ANSWERS

Activity 1.1: Reflective Practice

The introduction of lockdown measures during the first wave of the COVID-19 pandemic (prior to the development of vaccines) is a complex public health intervention that just about all of us have been affected by. Some countries such as Korea managed to avoid lockdown in this phase of the pandemic because they had learnt from the Middle East Respiratory Syndrome (MERS) and had well-developed test-and-trace services.

The problem lockdown measures were addressing was the community spread of the COVID-19 virus and the potential for health services to become overwhelmed. Full or partial lockdown was implemented when earlier interventions such as containment and test and trace had failed to prevent widespread community transmission.

The planned actions for lockdown during the pandemic varied by time and country but included one or more of the following:

- Encouragement of those with pre-existing conditions (and therefore at higher risk of infection) to shield, which meant avoiding leaving the house or having anyone inside their house.
- Enforcement of stay-at-home rules with minimal opportunities for meeting other people.
- Self-isolation for those who became infected.
- Shutting of non-essential shops and services, schools and workplaces.
- Social distancing in public spaces, such as supermarkets.
- Wearing of face masks in public spaces.

The change it was intended to make (e.g. the outcomes) were:

1. A reduction in overall community transmission of the virus and subsequently a reduction in the number of infections.
2. A reduction in more serious cases of COVID-19 which resulted in hospital admissions, an increase in intensive care beds, and pressure on health care services.
3. A reduction in household transmission.

Was it well developed?

This was an unusual situation as many countries such as the United Kingdom (UK) and the United States of America (USA) had not recently encountered a public health problem of the magnitude of the epidemic. Because of the urgency of the situation, planned activities were developed based *not only* on best scientific evidence and expert opinion but also on political and socioeconomic considerations. It could be argued that many of the lessons learnt from outbreaks of other, similar viruses (e.g. Severe Acute Respiratory Syndrome (SARS), Middle East Respiratory Syndrome (MERS)) were not applied. Decisions to implement a full or partial lockdown were largely based on non-health considerations (e.g. political and socioeconomic factors).

Did it create the anticipated change?

The answer here is yes, but the magnitude of the effect depended on a number of factors. In some countries such as New Zealand, the lockdown was very successful, whereas in other countries such as the USA it was less so. The factors that affected success included: public compliance and government enforcement; political will; public health capacity and surveillance systems; health systems capacity; and border control. In this list, you may notice that some of these factors can be grouped together, perhaps into *context* (political will and compliance) and *systems* (healthcare and surveillance). These are incredibly important issues to consider in developing any intervention and we will be referring to them throughout the book.

2
PRINCIPLES OF INTERVENTION DEVELOPMENT

Learning objectives

After reading this chapter, you will be able to:

- Understand the principles to be considered in intervention development
- Use these principles to plan the foundation of your intervention from the outset
- Understand the importance and role of co-production in intervention development.

Scenario 2.1

Smoking cessation intervention

Aziz has just started in his role as public health officer. He has been asked to look at a report about a pilot smoking intervention and present a summary of whether it was successful or not. His boss wants to know whether they should continue to fund it and has asked him to prepare a presentation for the weekly team meeting. He examines the report which includes statistics on the uptake of the intervention; the demographics of who participated; the number of people who stopped smoking; the demographics of those who stopped smoking; and what resources were needed to deliver it. There are also comments from those receiving the intervention and those delivering the intervention.

Which data should Aziz focus on in his presentation? What would define the success of this intervention?

INTRODUCTION

Following on from the scenario above, take a moment to think about what you would consider to be a successful intervention. For many people, the first thing they might think is that it needs to be effective. But would it still be successful if it was effective yet it increased health inequalities? Or what about if it was effective but unacceptable to the population? Or effective but caused harm? Or was so expensive that it was not sustainable? Or what about if the healthcare workers you want to deliver the intervention are unable to because of lack of time and other commitments? In intervention development, you need to consider all of these issues. A successful intervention is one which is effective, acceptable, sustainable, implementable and equitable. Or put another way, a successful intervention is one which creates significant and positive lasting change for those who will benefit from it most.

Table 2.1 outlines the principles which will be discussed in this chapter, which will help to ensure that your intervention is successful in all the aspects mentioned above. These principles underpin the intervention development process, and as such comprise the foundations of a good intervention. Some of these you may innately use already but you can increase success by being more conscious and transparent in your decision making. We will return to these principles frequently as we progress through this book. By the end of this book, our goal is that the principles outlined in Table 2.1 will have become engrained in your thinking and practice.

Table 2.1   Nine principles of intervention development

Key focus	Principle
1. Need	Understand the population with whom you intend to receive your intervention, the problem you will be intervening in, and the context in which you will be intervening
2. Health inequalities	Ensure that your intervention will not widen health inequalities
3. Ethics	Ensure that your intervention is ethical and will not cause harm
4. Assets	Take an assets-based approach to intervention development
5. Sustainability	Build sustainability into your intervention
6. Systems	Understand and consider the influence of systems in relation to the context in which you intend to implement your intervention
7. Evaluation	Consider development and evaluation together: Evaluation is best planned at the time of intervention development
8. Transparent reporting	Record sufficient information to facilitate transparent reporting of your process
9. Iterative process	Develop your intervention using an iterative process

Principle 1. Identify the need for an intervention

To effectively develop an intervention that will work for your population, it is important to be able to demonstrate the need for the intervention to the individuals or populations who will receive it. This seems obvious but it is an important point to make explicit. One of the mistakes that professionals often make is assuming that the needs they perceive as important are the same as what the community perceives. Trying to impose a solution for a need that is not recognised by the local community or population is likely to result in low adherence and uptake.

Knowledge link: This topic is also covered in Chapter 4

Principle 2. Ensure that your intervention will not widen health inequalities

Health inequalities refer to unfair differences in health outcomes between different groups within the population. Health inequalities have been demonstrated across income, ethnicity, race, gender, disability, sexual orientation and social class. These factors have also been shown to interact with one another (intersectionality). **Socioeconomic status** is one of the terms you will hear frequently in the literature related to health inequalities. This generally refers to income, education and occupation. Life expectancy is often used as an indicator of the presence of health inequalities. For example, the number of years that someone can expect to live has been shown to vary by geographical region, with those living in areas of poverty living shorter lives than those in areas that are more financially well off. The main social pathways and mechanisms through which social determinants affect people's health can usefully be seen through three perspectives: (1) social selection or social mobility; (2) social causation; and (3) life course perspectives (World Health Organisation, 2010). This is relevant to intervention development because the act of intervening may inadvertently widen health inequalities (White et al., 2009). This phenomenon is known as 'intervention-generated inequality'. An intervention has the potential to produce or increase inequalities if it has one or more of the features shown in Figure 2.1.

Knowledge link: This topic is also covered in Chapters 4 and 6

Specifically, interventions are likely to increase inequalities if they are more accessible to, adopted more frequently by, adhered to more closely by or are more effective in individuals, groups or populations which have more resources or education (Veinot et al., 2018). These are also the population groups which may receive the least benefit from the intervention because they often have lower risk factors than those with less income or education. This is why some interventions (sometimes referred to as targeted interventions) are specifically developed with and for populations who have higher levels of risk factors or fewer resources and assets.

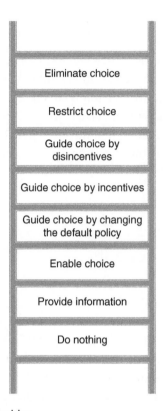

Figure 2.1   The intervention ladder

Interventions which use technology, such as health informatics and digital devices, are particularly prone to increasing health inequalities. Veinot et al. (2018) described how health technology interventions increased inequalities through assessing them against the four critiera:

(i) Is there equal accessibility of health technology by all members of the community? No. Information technologies are disproportionately available to those with higher incomes, to educated, young and urban populations.

(ii) Are they equally adopted by the population? No. Online mental health and substance use interventions are adopted more frequently by people with higher incomes and education, even though these conditions are more prevalent among those with a lower income and education.

(iii) Do they have the same level of adherence? No. People with less formal education are more likely to drop out of a health technology intervention after trying it.

(iv) Are they equally effective? No. Whilst the efficacy may be similar, effectiveness may be impaired by three factors: poor access, adoption or adherence.

It is worth pointing out that in some cases mobile phone technology is proving to be a huge asset and can help reduce health inequalities. There are a number of interventions in low- and middle-income countries which use mobile phones very successfully to support health and other outcomes. Similarly, there is evidence that most homeless people have mobile phones so these can be used to reach them for health services. So, whilst in some cases technology can widen health inequalities, in other situations it can be used as a potential solution.

There are a number of resources you can use to design your intervention or activity to have maximum effect in reducing health inequalities. One example is the Health Inequalities Assessment Toolkit (HIAT) (Porroche-Escudero and Popay, 2020). You can also consider whether your intervention is likely to cause inequalities in access, adoption or adherence. Essentially, you are mitigating a potentially unethical intervention which could, at its worst, produce harm to a community, which is the focus of our next principle.

Principle 3. Ensure that your intervention is ethical and will not cause harm

When we talk about **ethics** in relation to interventions, we are talking about a system of moral principles which we use to guide our decision making as we navigate the process of intervention development. We apply these moral principles to avoid creating harm. However, morals are neither static nor universal – what is morally acceptable in one decade or country may be morally unacceptable (and therefore unethical) in another time or place. One of the central issues is whether public health initiatives are compatible with the concept of respect for individual autonomy. Individual choice is grounded in the theory of liberalism and implies that individual rights are paramount. However, many public health policies, such as health screening and smoking bans, are grounded in utilitarian positions and based on outcomes such as a reduction in population levels of cancer and smoking. Thus, there may be a tension between a policy aimed at the benefit of the population, and other policies or interventions which promote individual autonomous decision making. Population public health, with its grounding in utilitarianism, is by nature paternalistic, in that it acts *'for the public good'* with little consultation with individuals. It has been contended that public health has expanded its remit to include controlling, or attempting to control, the choices, or even the desires, of human beings. Whether you agree or disagree with this argument, you may need to consider how much restriction of choice your population is prepared to accept for a population health benefit that they may not experience. This argument was evident during the lockdown phase of the COVID-19 pandemic in some countries. Large sections of the population were prepared to forgo some of their civil liberties to prevent the spread of the virus to vulnerable groups.

Knowledge link: This topic is also covered in Chapters 6 and 7

However, others felt that it was an infringement of their civil liberties and took to the streets to protest about the wearing of masks, quarantine and social distancing.

The UK Nuffield Council on Bioethics provides a detailed intervention ladder to illustrate the potential for such harms, with interventions at population levels (policies and laws) posing greater ethical challenges than those at individual levels (such as individual behaviour change interventions) (Figure 2.1) (Nuffield Council on Bioethics, 2007). The Council argues that public health interventions are often seen as infringing individual liberties, particularly when they involve an element of coercion or enforcement. Another example is smoking cessation interventions. Interventions can take place at the population level through legislation to ban smoking in public places as well as at community and individual levels (e.g. provision of stop smoking services). At the population level, the introduction of legislation to ban smoking in public places eliminates choice, but may achieve a greater reduction in lung disease and health inequalities.

Since complex public health problems usually require intervention at multiple levels, it is essential to consider ethical implications at each level of intervention to ensure that the intervention is ethically sound and acceptable. You should think through the potential harms that may be caused either directly or indirectly by your intervention. You may wish to include an ethical review of your intervention involving an external party who can look at your intervention plans to help you identify and understand any potential ethical issues. Involving stakeholders in co-production of the intervention will also help you to gauge the ethics of the intervention. It is important to remember that public health policies (and interventions) should use the least intrusive means to achieve the required public health benefit.

Knowledge link:
This topic is
also covered in
Chapters 5, 6
and 7

It is also worth noting in this section (and we will return to this issue in later sections of the book that, depending on the politics of both national and local government, some very effective interventions may be seen as politically undesirable or unpalatable. For example, poverty is one of the main determinants of ill health. Most governments are aware of this, but very few do everything within their power to improve the financial position of their poorest citizens as they fear that it would be politically damaging. Instead, resources are often funnelled into individual-level interventions which are often more resource intensive, less effective and can increase inequalities. Some countries and funding bodies are working to change this focus on individual-level intervention, and there have been some more promising interventions to reduce poverty. One such intervention is the basic income – a regular payment that goes to everyone, regardless of personal circumstance.

Principle 4: Take an assets-based approach

Assets are essentially the resources of an individual, a community or a system that can be utilised to increase the acceptability, sustainability and effectiveness of the intervention. They include:

- Human resources such as staff capacity, skills, enthusiasm, motivation and experience
- Economic resources such as funding and capital
- Physical assets such as empty rooms and buildings
- Community assets such as local groups and businesses
- Geographical assets such as beaches, parks, areas of shared space, derelict or unused land
- Cultural assets such as faith-based or art communities and spaces.

These assets will increase the likelihood of success of an intervention in several ways. First, any intervention is likely to need some resources. If these resources (assets) are available in the local setting, then the overall costs of the intervention can be reduced. Second, using community or individual assets can create a feeling of ownership of the intervention. For example, rather than training people in a certain skill, you may find that those skills are already there, and people are proud to use them. Third, they are more likely to increase the sustainability of the intervention. This is because you are not trying to find continued funding for external resources such as individuals to deliver the intervention, and so on. One of the major issues with any new intervention is that funding is achieved for only a short period, and after that period the intervention is unsustainable.

Knowledge link: This topic is also covered in Chapter 6

Whilst developing your intervention, it is useful to take stock of existing assets and think about how these might be utilised in intervention development. This is best achieved by consulting with your stakeholders. You may want to develop an assets map.

Principle 5. Build sustainability into your intervention

One of the most common comments we hear from communities and practitioners is that they had a great service or activity a few years ago but it stopped when funding ran out. They are often reluctant to engage with any further interventions because they think the same thing will happen again. This happens because **sustainability**, that is, durability, has not been considered in the developmental phase.

Knowledge link: This topic is also covered in Chapter 7

Sustainability is usually a direct consequence of the extent to which an intervention is embedded within the systems and routines in which it operates (Proctor et al., 2011). The last thing you want to happen is for you and others to invest effort into the development of an intervention that will not last in the long term. Ideally, you are looking to create something which will be sustainable for many years and therefore contribute to positive outcomes in the months and years to come. As we pointed out, an unsustainable intervention can also affect the morale of the participants involved and result in them being less likely to engage with such interventions again. As noted in our ethics principle, this is a harm and should be anticipated and mitigated against.

A systematic review identified eight critical factors influencing the sustainability of health-promotion interventions (Bodkin and Hakimi, 2020). These were broadly defined as:

(i)   organisational capacity (i.e. resources, staffing, etc.) [see Principle 4];

(ii) partnerships developed through co-production and a high level of involvement to ensure a sense of ownership;

(iii) strategic planning in terms of embedding the intervention within existing structures, routines and processes;

(iv) funding;

(v)   fit/alignment in terms of the extent to which the intervention aligns with community need, community priorities, community opinion and, if occurring within an organisation, that organisation's core mandate and day-to-day operations;

(vi) ongoing evaluation since it is essential to demonstrate the effectiveness or otherwise of the intervention in order to justify its implementation over time;

(vii) capacity building, which refers to whether the intervention presents opportunities for individuals to grow, particularly if those opportunities offer transferable skills;

(viii) an intervention champion defined as a named and influential person within the organisation or community, who essentially advocates for the needs of the intervention.

Principle 6. Understand and consider the influence of systems in relation to your intervention

Knowledge link: This topic is also covered in Chapter 3

Interventions should be viewed not as sets of decontextualised activities, but as 'events' within complex social systems. The term system can be used to describe a wide array of phenomena. For example, from a social science perspective, systems may range from a family to a neighbourhood, an organisation, a school district or the national welfare system. Within the context of intervention development, a system is the set of actors, activities and settings that are directly or indirectly perceived to have influence in, or be affected by, the intervention. For example, a speed reduction intervention to reduce traffic accidents is not implemented in a vacuum, but in the wider traffic system. This traffic system may have a large number of other interventions which may either complement or compete with the intervention. These include activities to increase traffic flow, reduce congestion, promote cycling and walking or encourage public transport. In another example, an intervention to increase free school meals for school children living in remote areas needs to consider not only the school system, but also the local food system and perhaps even local transport systems.

Chapter 3

Principle 7. Consider development and evaluation together: Evaluation is best planned at the time of intervention development

Intervention development is closely linked with evaluation and they should be considered together. It is necessary to consider evaluation from the outset. Throughout this book, we refer to evaluation using a definition used by the World Health Organisation and United Nations Evaluation Group (UNEG) (World Health Organisation, 2021). This definition states that:

Knowledge link:
This topic is
also covered in
Chapter 9

> An evaluation is an assessment, as systematic and impartial as possible of an activity, project, programme, strategy, policy, theme, sector, operational area or institutional per-formance. It focuses on expected and achieved accomplishments examining the results chain, processes, contextual factors and causality, in order to understand achievements or the lack thereof. It aims at determining the relevance, impact, effectiveness, efficiency and sustainability of the interventions and contributions of the organizations of the UN system.

As you progress through the 6SQuID steps, you will eventually learn how to plan a **logic model**, which is essentially a chain of activities, outputs and outcomes that is central to your intervention. You will also learn how to trigger those outcomes by applying carefully thought-out activities. In order to determine whether your intervention is effective, you should specify how you will measure and/or assess:

Knowledge link:
This topic is
also covered in
Chapter 6

- each of the outcomes in your outcomes chain
- what data are currently available/collected to measure your outcomes
- what new data you would need to collect
- delivery and implementation of the intervention.

Knowledge link:
This topic is
also covered in
Chapter 7

General statements about effectiveness and ineffectiveness are necessary but not sufficient in and of themselves. You should outline how you plan to explore why your intervention has had its effect, whether there are elements of it that were more effective than others, whether there are specific groups of people who it worked best for and what could be improved or refined. These questions should be considered alongside the development process.

Another reason to plan evaluation alongside developmental work is that it can be easy to lose sight of the available resources as you develop your intervention. The majority of interventions have finite resources, and these costs need to be divided amongst staffing pay, travel, consumables, and intervention expenses, in addition to evaluation. These can add up quickly. It is therefore necessary to set aside evaluation costs prior to intervention implementation, to 'protect' these costs from being used elsewhere.

Principle 8. Record sufficient information to facilitate transparent reporting of your process

It is good practice to record as much information about your process and findings as possible. You should aim to provide sufficient detail that someone could replicate the intervention elsewhere. You should provide as much detail as possible about each of the activities involved and how these relate to your causal factors and eventual anticipated outcomes. If you have followed steps 1–4 of the 6SQuID framework, you will naturally have gathered the information that you need to report your process and findings transparently.

Imagine that you are developing an intervention to reduce substance use in your local community. Someone comes to you and says that they have just finished evaluating an intervention in their own local community focusing upon the same problem. The evaluation showed that the intervention was effective in reducing substance use by 20%. The first questions you would ask would likely be along the lines of the following. What precisely did you do to achieve that? What would I need to do to achieve a similar result in my own community? Can you walk me through each step of your intervention? Failure to provide sufficient information as to what you did in your intervention means that others cannot replicate (and therefore benefit from) what you achieved. This situation is like providing someone with a pill to cure an illness, discovering it works and then being unable to describe the ingredients of that pill so that others can benefit. Using the same example, you should also be curious as to which causal factors are being targeted by this successful intervention. This is important because you would want to know whether the factors contributing to the problem in the case of the successful intervention are the same causal factors that are contributing to the problem in your local community. If these are not the same, then it is unlikely that this intervention will work for you since they are targeting factors that are irrelevant/less important to the problem in your local community.

Guidance and frameworks exist to facilitate the transparent reporting of interventions. For example, the TiDieR-PHP reporting guidelines for population health and policy interventions advise that intervention developers report: the rationale behind the intervention, including how intervention activities are linked to the expected effects upon causal factors and outcomes, what materials are used, how the intervention was planned and delivered, who provided it, where it was provided, when and how often it was provided and aspects of its delivery, such as how well it was delivered (Campbell et al., 2018).

Principle 9. Develop your intervention using an iterative and dynamic process

The steps to intervention development outlined in this book are not linear. There may be points along the way when you need to return to previous steps. For example, during the testing phase of your intervention (Step 5), you may discover issues with the activities underpinning your intervention which require reconsideration of your theory of action (i.e. a return to Step 4), followed by further testing. Progression to later steps should not prevent you from returning to steps that you have already visited along your intervention journey.

In thinking through your intervention, there are points at which questions are raised that require you to revisit steps. As you navigate this book, you will see that each step raises new questions that need to be addressed to optimise your intervention. Sometimes the answers to these questions will cause you to revisit work on previous steps. This is healthy and is a sign of good practice. Intervention development needs to be properly thought through. A linear process does not facilitate the type of flexible thinking required to do this.

The value of co-production and team working

Co-production is a core feature of community engagement and involvement and helps to ensure that health research contributes to building knowledge and generating innovations that benefit users of research (Tembo et al., 2021). The key to an effective, acceptable, sustainable, implementable and equitable intervention is working closely with those who receive the intervention; and those stakeholders who are involved in funding, delivery or implementation. We would encourage you, as far as possible, to view intervention development as a team activity in which everyone is seen as having a role in defining the problem and contributing towards the solution. Co-production can be defined as an approach in which researchers, practitioners and the public work together, sharing power and responsibility from the start to the end of the project, including the generation of knowledge (Bortoli, 2021). It is generally agreed that research is enhanced by the inclusion of experiential expertise and that subsequent research is better informed by community preferences and needs (Collins and Evans, 2002; Fischer, 2000). As definitions and approaches to co-production may vary, it is useful to consider these four pillars to ensure meaningful involvement (Pennington et al., 2018):

1. Power is agreed and acknowledged as being held jointly by all people involved.
2. There is active and full involvement in all decisions that impact upon the project and evaluation of its success.
3. Potential barriers to access and participation (including income, education, gender, ethnicity, age, disability, language and caring responsibilities) are acknowledged and tackled.
4. When appropriate and desired by the community, there is full and active involvement in implementation of the solutions.

Co-production is underpinned by four principles of equality, diversity, access and reciprocity. Briefly in this context, equality means that everyone is an equal partner, deserving of mutual respect, and involved in all stages of the intervention development and evaluation process, including decision making. Diversity means that a range of partners are involved, from the people who are affected by the problem, to those who are implementing or funding the intervention. Access refers to being able to be part of the process regardless of disability, childcare issues or other barriers to participation, including financial issues. And reciprocity means that people get something back for putting something in. This could range from financial rewards for participation, to the feeling of ownership, and contributing to solving a problem for their community. Each individual or partnership organization will have their own reason for wanting to be involved, and it is important to understand what they want out of the process from the outset.

Engaging and co-producing your intervention with your population and key stakeholders from the beginning of its development will increase its effectiveness and acceptability. For example, if your goal is to get your workforce to eat more healthily during the working day you will need to engage with them to ensure that any proposed solutions are acceptable. After all, would you make a cup of tea for someone before first asking if they take milk or sugar? You might do, but they probably wouldn't like it, or at worst, wouldn't drink it. They might not even like tea, and in the worst case scenario they may be allergic to cow's milk. This also holds true of interventions. You will also need to engage with the manager and catering staff to ensure that your intervention is practical in terms of the resources available to them. Similarly, in terms of evaluation, stakeholders can provide valuable information about which designs and data collection methods are likely to be feasible given the context; which outcomes are likely to be most appropriate and achievable; and how best to gather data.

Knowledge link:
This topic is
also covered in
Chapter 9

Your goal is not only to develop an effective and acceptable intervention, but also to implement and embed your intervention within its intended context to maximise the likelihood of its success. For example, an intervention to increase healthcare worker hand-hygiene behaviour that demands high resources in terms of time may not work very well in time-intensive environments such as intensive care units. Such an intervention might work better in less time-intensive healthcare environments like care of the elderly wards. Knowing the constraints of delivery and implementation can help you to develop your intervention accordingly.

Knowledge link:
This topic is
also covered in
Chapter 7

In short, co-production is fundamental to intervention development. Without it, your intervention is unlikely to reach its full potential. Throughout the remainder of this book, we refer to co-production frequently, and provide advice on how to do this effectively at all stages of the intervention development process. We will begin, however, with some steps as to how to decide on who to partner with, and how to begin establishing relationships.

Identifying your partners, creating a team and developing relationships

Developing an intervention team should start as early as possible. The first step is to identify partners who are likely to be the key stakeholders, and others that can play a role in creating lasting and effective change. This is likely to be an iterative process, in that you may not be aware of all your partners and stakeholders at the beginning of the process. You should also be prepared for the team to change over time, with new partnerships forming as the process develops and new insights are gained. Some of the stakeholders you could include, the role they can play in intervention development and how their involvement may benefit them, are described in Table 2.2 and in more detail below.

Table 2.2 Potential roles for stakeholders in the intervention development process

Stakeholders	Role in the process	Benefit to them
Individuals affected by the problem	Understanding the need, defining the problem and its causes	Feelings of empowerment and ownership
	Identifying potential health inequalities, ethical issues, and assets	Developing skills in teamworking
		Giving back to their community
	Understanding barriers to uptake and acceptability of solutions. Possible role in delivery of the intervention (e.g. peer support)	Self-esteem and confidence as a result of being heard and taking part in decisions which affect their community
		Financial (if this is an option, community members should be paid for their time)
		Inclusion on a CV
Organisations representing those affected by the problem, vulnerable groups or seldom heard groups	Understanding the need, defining the problem and its causes	Supporting their community
	Identifying potential health inequalities, ethical issues, assets and systems	Being listened to
		Recognition of their expertise and the importance of their organisational knowledge
	Potential role in funding, delivery, sustainability, and evaluation of the intervention	Possible solutions and associated resources for their community
	Identifying sources of data that could be used in the evaluation	
Experts	Understanding the need, defining the problem and its causes	Job satisfaction
	Identifying potential health inequalities, ethical issues, assets and systems	Networks
		Skill building
	Potential role in funding, delivery, sustainability, and evaluation of the intervention	
	Identifying sources of data that could be used in the evaluation	
Funders and/or those involved in resourcing the intervention	Role in funding, delivery, sustainability and evaluation of the intervention	Efficient and effective use of scarce resources
	Identifying sources of data that could be used in the evaluation	

(Continued)

Table 2.2 (Continued)

Stakeholders	Role in the process	Benefit to them
Decision makers and policy makers	Understanding the need, defining the problem and its causes	New solutions for difficult problems
	Identifying potential health inequalities, ethical issues, assets, competing or complementary policies and systems	
	Understanding the policy landscape and opportunities and threats for the intervention	
	Role in developing solutions that fit with current or future policies or guidelines	
	Potential role in funding, delivery, sustainability and evaluation of the intervention	
	Identifying sources of data that could be used in the evaluation	
People who represent the different systems	Identifying potential health inequalities, ethical issues, assets, competing or complementary policies and systems	New solutions for difficult problems
	Potential role in developing innovative solutions, funding, delivery, sustainability and evaluation of the intervention	
	Identifying sources of data that could be used in the evaluation	
Those responsible for delivery of the intervention	Identifying potential health inequalities, ethical issues, assets, competing or complementary policies and systems	Having a voice in decisions often made by others that impact on their workload
	Understanding how any intervention developed will compete or interact with other programmes or policies, or features of the system, including resources, time and physical space	Supporting their local community

Job satisfaction |

Individuals or representatives of groups who are affected by the problem

This includes a range of people who experience and/or are affected by the problem either directly or indirectly. For example, if you are wanting to develop an intervention to look at how to increase female empowerment in rural communities in Pakistan, you may want to include women of different ages, and with different family or community roles. If you are looking to reduce alcohol-related harm in young people, you may want to include young people, parents and community members.

Organisations representing those affected by the problem, vulnerable groups or seldom heard groups

Sometimes it is difficult to involve those directly affected by the problem. In this case, individuals or organisations who represent such groups could be considered stakeholders. For example, people with advanced dementia may not be able to participate fully, so a group representing their needs may be more appropriate. Where possible, it is always preferable to have the people directly affected by the problem involved.

Experts

People who have training and expertise specifically related to the problem area can bring a valuable perspective. These could be researchers or practitioners who might have considerable experience of either the problem or potential solutions.

Funders or those responsible for resourcing any intervention

If your intervention is likely to include any sort of resources, you will need to think about who may be involved in paying or providing the resources in the short, medium and longer term. As you may not know what resources are required at the beginning of the process, it may be difficult to identify these stakeholders. However, if you are working in a health board or government area then you will want to involve someone who has responsibility for resource allocation, or at least have someone that can provide input on these issues. There may also be industry partners you wish to involve in the team who can provide you with technology resources.

Decision makers and policy makers

Those involved in policy decision making in the community or region, or even the country, could be invited to be part of the intervention development team. This could be quite strategic because of their influence in the decision-making process and the capacity they may have to influence change. Involving these individuals can also create a feeling of ownership over the final product and ensure that it fits with other priorities and activities taking place.

People who represent the different systems

These individuals may not be obvious at the beginning of the intervention development process, and may need to be added to your team as you work through the six steps. However, your understanding of the problem might identify some of these partners. For example, if the problem is a derelict and unsafe park, you may need to include someone who is responsible for park maintenance. As you begin to develop your intervention, you may realise there are other people you wish to involve such as city planners and the police.

Those responsible for delivery of the intervention

Again, these individuals may not be obvious from the outset, but at some stage in intervention development you will need to include people who your co-production team may want to be responsible for delivering or implementing the services. If you know who these people are, it is useful to involve them as soon as possible. They can provide an understanding of how any intervention developed will compete or interact with other programmes or policies, or features of the system including resources, time and physical space. For example, you may want to develop an alcohol brief intervention to be delivered by midwives to pregnant women. Having midwives on the team will ensure that it is deliverable within the consultation period, and will not be at the expense of other important activities such as assessing the risk of domestic abuse.

Developing the intervention team

Once you have decided on an initial list of stakeholders, the next step is to develop the intervention team comprising of you and your team (if you have one), and the stakeholders. An understanding of how teams work is beneficial, as this illustrates the stages of team development and where the potential difficulties may lie. Figure 2.2 shows an example of a team development ladder which you may find useful in making the most of the interactions you have.

In conjunction with the ladder, you can also consider the five-stage development process that some teams follow to become successful. This was developed by Bruce Tuckman, an educational psychologist and categorised as the forming, storming, norming, performing and adjourning stages (Tuckman, 1965; Tuckman and Jensen, 1977). Team progress through the stages is shown in Figure 2.3. Each of these will be considered in relation to intervention development.

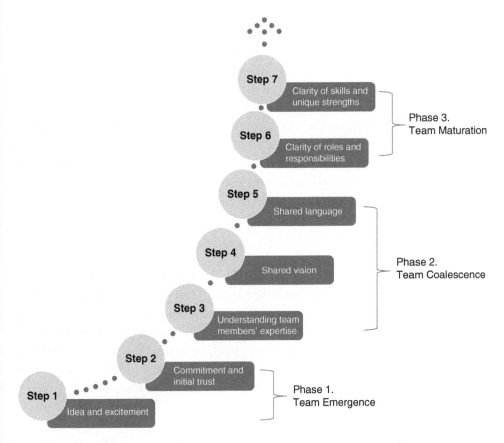

Figure 2.2   Developing your team

Source: Cross et al. (2019). Reproduced by kind permission of the authors.

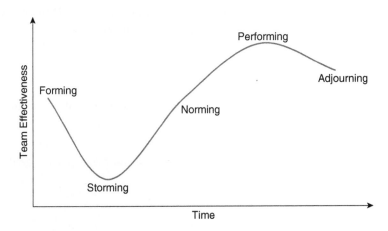

Figure 2.3   Most high-performing teams go through five stages of team development

Source: John/Lynn Bruton and Lumen Learning (n.d.). (CC BY)

Forming stage

The forming stage involves a period of understanding the purpose of the team and the project, and getting acquainted. Uncertainty is high during this stage, and people are looking for leadership and authority. Team members may ask questions to themselves such as 'What does the team offer me?' 'What is expected of me?' 'Will I fit in?' Most interactions are social as members get to know each other. This will likely happen during the first meeting you have with the team. Developing relationships is very important at this stage. It is best to try and get everyone together either face to face or via video-conferencing, which typically works better than telephone. You can use the initial meeting to generate excitement and ideas, gain commitment and explain each team member's unique expertise.

Storming stage

The storming stage is the most difficult and critical stage to pass through. It is a period potentially marked by conflict and competition as individual personalities emerge. Members may disagree on the vision or the nature of the problem being considered. To get through this stage, the team should work to overcome obstacles, accept individual differences and work through conflicting ideas to try and reach solutions that address issues such as health inequalities or the needs of those who are most affected. This stage presents an opportunity to work with any differences that arise to arrive at new understandings.

Norming stage

During the norming stage, group consensus begins to develop a vision for the work that will be undertaken, including clarifying the problem and potential solutions. The team should begin forming trust, a shared vision and a common language. Differences begin to be resolved at this stage, and a sense of cohesion and unity emerges.

Performing stage

In the performing stage, consensus and cooperation have been well established and the team is well functioning. There is a clear and stable structure, and members are committed to the team's mission. Problems and conflicts may emerge, but they are dealt with constructively. The team is focused on problem solving and meeting team goals.

Adjourning stage

In the adjourning stage, most of the team's goals have been accomplished. The emphasis is on wrapping up final tasks and documenting the effort and results. There may be some regrets as the work undertaken by the team ends, so a ceremonial acknowledgement of the work and success of the team can be helpful. This is likely to be after you have reached step 6 of 6SQuID. However, you may find that the group has worked so well together that they go on to develop other interventions within the community, with some members leaving and others joining.

Team norms and cohesiveness

Think of a time when you were part of a team. How did you know how to act? How did you know what behaviours were acceptable or what level of performance was required? Teams develop **norms** that guide the activities of team members. Team norms set a standard for behaviour, attitude and performance that all team members are expected to follow. Norms are rules that are implicitly understood by all team members. They are not always written down. Norms are effective because each team member wants to support the team as a whole and preserve relationships. As mentioned previously, co-production has its own set of approaches and principles that will guide teamwork. These approaches and principles should in time become team norms. As you might expect, the team leader (possibly yourself!) plays an important part in establishing productive norms by acting as role models.

Activity 2.1

Teamwork

You want to bring together a group of stakeholders to help you develop an intervention to address youth unemployment in a low-income neighbourhood. Who would you invite to the group and why?

We will return to team development in subsequent chapters of the book.

Tools for co-production and intervention development

Throughout this book, we present a range of tools you can use for intervention development and co-production. Although some of these are in specific chapters, we encourage you to use them where and when you think they fit best into your own unique intervention development process.

SUMMARY

This chapter has outlined and described nine principles related to intervention development. The principles should serve as a foundation as you start to build your intervention. These are to:

1. understand the population with whom you intend to receive your intervention, the problem you will be intervening upon, and the context in which you will be intervening; work closely throughout the development process with those who receive your intervention and key stakeholders;
2. ensure that your intervention will not widen health inequalities;
3. ensure that your intervention is ethical and will not cause harm;
4. take an assets-based approach to intervention development;
5. build sustainability into your intervention;
6. understand and consider the influence of systems in relation to your intervention;
7. consider development and evaluation together;
8. record sufficient information to facilitate transparent reporting of your process; and
9. develop your intervention using an iterative process.

Co-production is the foundation of intervention development and will help you to address these principles. Keep these principles in mind as you make your way through the chapters. Adherence to these principles will ensure that your intervention is more likely to be acceptable, sustainable and successful.

FURTHER READING

Frerichs, F., Hassmiller Lich, K., Dave, G., and Corbie-Smith, G. (2016) 'Integrating systems science and community-based participatory research to achieve health equity', *American Journal of Public Health,* 106: 215–22. https://doi.org/10.2105/AJPH.2015.302944

World Health Organisation (2010) *A Conceptual Framework for Action on the Social Determinants of Health.* Discussion Paper. Geneva: WHO Document Production Services. www.who.int/social_determinants/corner/SDHDP2.pdf?ua=1

REFERENCES

Bodkin, A., and Hakimi, S. (2020) 'Sustainable by design: a systematic review of factors for health promotion program sustainability', *BMC Public Health, 20:* 964.

Bortoli, S. (2021). *Guidance on Co-Producing a Research Project.* London: NIHR.

Bruton, J., Bruton, L., and Lumen Learning (n.d.) 'The five stages of team development'. https://courses.lumenlearning.com/suny-principlesmanagement/chapter/reading-the-five-stages-of-team-development, accessed 11 June 2021.

Campbell, M., Katikireddi, S. V., Hoffmann, T., Armstrong, R., Waters, E., and Craig, P. (2018) 'TIDieR-PHP: a reporting guideline for population health and policy interventions', *BMJ*, 16 May; 361: k1079. doi: 10.1136/bmj.k1079. PMID: 29769210; PMCID: PMC5954974.

Collins, H. M., and Evans, R. (2002) 'The third wave of science studies: studies of expertise and experience', *Social Studies of Science*, 32 (2): 235–96. doi:10.1177/0306312702032002003

Cross, J. E., Love, H., and Fisher, E. (2019) 'I'm ready, are you ready? How do you know if your team is ready?', Science of Team Science (SciTS) Conference, Lansing, MI, 20 May.

Fischer, F. (2000) *Citizens, Experts, and the Environment: The Politics of Local Knowledge.* Durham, NC: Duke University Press.

Hawe, P., Shiell, A., and Riley, T. (2009) 'Theorising interventions as events in systems', *American Journal of Community Psychology*, 43 (3–4): 267–76.

Nuffield Council on Bioethics (2007) *Public Health: Ethical Issues.* London: Nuffield Council on Bioethics. nuffieldbioethics.org, accessed 21 April 2021.

Pennington, A., Watkins, M., Bagnall, A.-M., South, J., and Corcoran, R. (2018) *A Systematic Review of Evidence on the Impacts of Joint Decision-Making on Community Wellbeing.* London: What Works Centre for Wellbeing.

Porroche-Escudero, A., and Popay, J. (2020) 'The Health Inequalities Assessment Toolkit: supporting integration of equity into applied health research', *Journal of Public Health*, fdaa047, https://doi.org/10.1093/pubmed/fdaa047

Proctor, E., Silmere, H., Raghavan, R., Hovmand, P., Aarons, G., Bunger, A., Griffey, R., and Hensley, M. (2011) 'Outcomes for implementation research: conceptual distinctions, measurement challenges, and research agenda', *Administration and Policy in Mental Health and Mental Health Services*, 38 (2): 65–76.

Tembo, D., Hickey, G., Montenegro, C., Chandler, D., Nelson, E., Porter, K., et al. (2021) 'Effective engagement and involvement with community stakeholders in the co-production of global health research', *BMJ*, 372: n178. doi:10.1136/bmj.n178

Tuckman, B. W. (1965) 'Developmental sequence in small groups', *Psychological Bulletin*, 63 (6): 384–99.

Tuckman, B. W., and Jensen, M. A. C. (1977) 'Stages of small-group development revisited', *Group & Organization Management, 2* (4): 419–27.

Veinot, T. C., Mitchell, H., and Ancker, J. S. (2018) 'Good intentions are not enough: how informatics interventions can worsen inequality', *Journal of the American Medical Informatics Association, 25* (8): 1080–8. https://doi.org/10.1093/jamia/ocy052

White, M., Adams, J., and Heywood, P. (2009) 'How and why do interventions that increase health overall widen inequalities within populations?', pp. 65–82 in S. Babones (ed.), *Social Inequality and Public Health.* Bristol: Policy Press.

World Health Organisation (WHO) (2010) *A Conceptual Framework for Action on the Social Determinants of Health.* Discussion Paper. Geneva: WHO Document Production Services.

World Health Organisation (2021) 'What we do: evaluation'. www.who.int/about/what-we-do/evaluation, accessed 9 May 2021.

ACTIVITY ANSWERS

Scenario 2.1: Smoking cessation intervention

Aziz needs to consider all aspects of success in his presentation, and make a judgement based on answers to the following questions:

1. Was it effective in reducing smoking? The number of people who successfully stopped smoking compared to when there was no intervention (or another intervention).
2. Was it acceptable? How high was uptake of the service and what did those who participated think of the service?
3. What was its impact on health inequalities? Were there differences, for example, in the age, gender, income and ethnicity of the people who stopped smoking?
4. Was it ethical? For example, were people pressurised or coerced into attending; was participation linked to welfare benefits or another benefit?
5. Was it equitable? Who had access to the service and participated in the service – were there differences in age, gender, income and ethnicity?
6. Was resource use acceptable given other constraints in the system? What resources were used, and were they taken away from other services (e.g. was a room needed that was normally used at the same time for a mother and baby clinic; was a health professional delivering the intervention at the time they normally provided home visits)?
7. Did it need adaptation? What were the views of those delivering and receiving the intervention? What changes were made, if any? Was it acceptable and workable in the longer term?
8. Was it sustainable? If it was taking resources away from other parts of the system, how would it be resourced in the future? What other services might be lost as a result?

Activity 2.1: Teamwork

You may consider inviting stakeholders for the reasons outlined in Table 2.3. It is important to note that this is not an exhaustive list.

Table 2.3   Potential reasons for inviting stakeholders (Activity 2.1 answer)

Stakeholder	Potential reasons
Employment services	Understanding of systems (their own and others such as social services)
	Could be involved with sustainability and delivery of intervention
	May know what has worked/not worked before
	Understanding of data available for evaluation
Employers: A range of small and larger employers in the area	Could be involved with intervention development, sustainability and delivery of some aspects of the intervention
	Identify assets in the area relating to unemployment

Stakeholder	Potential reasons
Young people who are unemployed	Input into understandings/decisions about acceptability, ethics, need, health inequalities
	Understanding of causal factors
	What would constitute success for young people
Representatives from schools and adult education	Understanding of services/education provided around employment. Understanding of some of the educational factors impacting on unemployment
	Could be involved with intervention development, sustainability and delivery of aspects of the intervention
Funders of services (e.g. employment, education)	Understanding of resources available for intervention development, and if the intervention was successful. May be essential to intervention sustainability if there are significant ongoing resources needed
Policy makers from employment, education, welfare, social services, health	Understanding of current and future policies and opportunities and threats for any interventions
	Understanding of how the intervention may link with similar interventions in other systems (such as a skills development programme for young people wanting to enter a health profession)
	Understanding of any routine data (such as unemployment statistics) that could be used in evaluating the success of the intervention
Youth groups and third-sector organisations	Understanding of local assets that could be used in the development of intervention
	Understanding of causal factors and what has/has not worked before
	Could be involved with intervention development, sustainability and delivery of aspects of the intervention

3
CAUSALITY, SYSTEMS AND COMPLEXITY

Learning objectives

After reading this chapter, you will:

- Understand the importance of causal relationships in intervention development and evaluation
- Understand what complexity means in terms of complex interventions
- Recognise the systems in which you are seeking to intervene
- Be able to distinguish between simple, complicated and complex approaches to intervention.

Scenario 3.1

Causal factors of headaches

Kieran has been having a lot of headaches recently, but rather than always taking medication he wants to see if he can prevent them. He has heard that some headaches are caused by dehydration, so he decided to drink a glass of water whenever his head starts to ache. Sometimes this prevents a full headache from developing, but not always. Next, Kieran wonders if his headaches happen at particular times, so he starts making a note on his calendar every time he starts to get a headache. Based on this information, he identifies that his headaches are more common in the afternoon and evening, but happen on various days of the week. So, he starts to add information to his calendar about whatever he has been doing before getting each headache. This reveals that the headaches happen when he has been working for long periods of time at his computer. He visits his optician who identifies that his eyesight has deteriorated so Kieran gets some new glasses, which help with the headaches. But Kieran still gets some headaches, so one of his friends suggests that he needs to add more screen breaks into his working day. This is difficult as Kieran often has back-to-back online meetings, so he talks to his line manager. His line manager has had similar health concerns raised by other employees so decides to reduce the number and length of meetings, meaning Kieran can go for brief walks during the day. His headaches are now much rarer. This scenario illustrates the importance of the way data are collected to understanding the causal factors (in this scenario, dehydration and excess screen time causing Kieran's headaches).

INTRODUCTION

In this chapter, we introduce and explain three concepts that are fundamental to current thinking about intervention development and evaluation: **causality, complexity** and **systems**. As we mentioned in Chapter 1, intervention is a *planned action* (or set of actions) that is designed to bring about a *desired change* (in one or more outcomes) in a defined population to address a social or health problem. Implied within this definition is the idea of cause and effect; without the intervention, one effect is expected to happen and with the intervention, a different effect is expected. For example, with no intervention your population may have a high incidence of lung cancer; with a law to prevent smoking in public places, you will see a reduction in incidence in lung cancer.

While there is a common understanding of the idea of cause and effect, there are also fields of science and philosophy devoted entirely to these topics. Consequently, we begin this chapter with a brief overview of what we mean in this book by causality and other terms such as determinants and risk factors. We will introduce the rationale for understanding these in the development and evaluation of interventions, which will be further developed in Chapters 4 and 9. Complexity and complex intervention approaches are explained before concluding this chapter with a discussion of systems and how we need to understand the relationships between different systems when we are embarking on intervention development and evaluation.

Knowledge link: This topic is also covered in Chapters 4 and 9

CAUSALITY

Understanding the causes of problems such as poor school attendance, loneliness or smoking is an essential part of intervention development and consequently part of the

Knowledge link:
This topic is
also covered in
Chapter 4

first 6SQuID step. Briefly, cause is what makes something else happen; effect refers to what happens afterwards (also referred to as the outcome). Simply put, cause refers to *why* something happened and effect to *what* happened. A single cause can have more than one effect, and a single effect (outcome) can have more than one cause. An example of a cause having more than one effect is cigarette smoking, which is a cause of lung cancer and other respiratory diseases. A single effect such as poor school attendance can be caused by factors such as bullying, lack of transport to school or disinterest in school. It is important at the start of intervention development to tease out all these potential causes and understand the way(s) that they may impact on the outcomes.

The term 'causation' or 'causality' has no single universal definition and the concept can be difficult to pin down (Parascandola and Weed, 2001). Parascandola and Weed (2001) distinguish between necessary and sufficient causes. Succinctly, a **necessary cause** is a causal factor without which the effect (outcome) cannot occur. For example, the lung condition asbestosis cannot occur without the inhalation of asbestos; asbestos is therefore a necessary cause of asbestosis. Tobacco smoking, on the other hand, is not a necessary cause of lung cancer. This is because lung cancer can occur in people who do not smoke. Neither asbestos nor smoking are sufficient causes for lung disease, as it is not certain that someone exposed to either chemical will develop this disease.

A **sufficient cause** is a casual factor with which the effect (outcome) must occur. Often, there are multiple components that together become a sufficient cause (sufficient-component causes), as in fire which occurs when there is a combination of heat, oxygen and fuel. When these three components come together, a fire will occur, but if any one of heat, oxygen or fuel is missing, the fire will not happen. Hence, understanding the causes starts to give you ideas about how to intervene to reduce a problem. To stop the fire, you will need to remove the heat, oxygen or fuel. Of course, most social interventions are not as simple as this, and many cannot put out a fire completely, only dampen the flames. As an example, a sufficient cause for AIDS might consist of the following components:

- infection with HIV
- significant deterioration of the immune system
- exposure to a pathogen that overcomes the weakened immune system, leading to an AIDS-defining illness.

The extent to which causes have different qualities of both necessity and sufficiency will inform the extent to which they are targets for intervention. For example, if a cause is both necessary and sufficient then intervening to remove that cause should prevent the outcome. So, a legal obligation to remove asbestos and not use asbestos in the future should prevent asbestosis. If a cause is neither necessary nor sufficient then intervening around that cause is unlikely to be effective. So, interventions to stop cigarette smoking (whether legislative or behavioural) will not prevent all cases of lung cancer (as not all lung cancer is caused by cigarette smoking). Most social instances of ill health have multiple causes, none of which are universally a necessary or sufficient cause of the behaviour, hence complex interventions often seek to address multiple components of this causal chain. Chapter 4 will explain in more detail how we identify the causes of the problem, and how to choose which cause(s) to focus our interventions on.

Knowledge link: This topic is also covered in Chapter 4

One of the most well-known examples from history is the establishment of the causal relationship between tobacco smoking and lung cancer. It was necessary for the researchers involved to provide evidence that tobacco smoke was causing lung cancer, and as part of this work a series of criteria was established. These were not intended to be a checklist, but attributes of causal relationships on which evidence could be gathered. The criteria are often known as the Bradford Hill criteria after Austin Bradford Hill who worked with Richard Doll in the UK to establish smoking as a cause of lung cancer (Hill, 1965).

Bradford Hill attributes of causal relationships

1. Strength or effect size: if the presence of a possible cause is found to be associated with a large increase in the outcome, this might be suggestive of a causal relationship.
2. Consistency or reproducibility: if multiple studies in different places with different populations find the same possible cause associated with the same outcome, this consistency or reproducibility is suggestive of a causal relationship.
3. Specificity: as discussed earlier, if the possible cause and outcome are specific to each other, as in many infectious diseases and their causative organism, it is more likely that you will have a necessary cause and consequently be able to detect stronger associations which suggest a causal relationship.
4. Temporality: it needs to be clear that the potential cause occurs before the outcome in order for the relationship to be causal.
5. Biological gradient or dose–response relationship: building on the first criteria, if the cause is something you can experience different doses of, like how much someone smokes, and higher doses are found to be associated with more of the outcome, this would seem to suggest a causal relationship.
6. Plausibility: is there a plausible mechanism by which the cause can lead to the effect? This is limited by the current state of knowledge.
7. Coherence: are different types of research on the same topic resulting in coherent findings?
8. Experiment: can you run an experiment or evaluation in a human sample to test the association?
9. Analogy: are there similar cause-and-effect relationships observed in animals and the laboratory?
10. Reversibility: if you can remove the cause and the outcome reduces then the relationship is more likely to be causal.

Interventions aim to interrupt, or break, a causal chain. If you intervene to prevent people from becoming infected with HIV, you can prevent them from developing AIDS. However, once someone is infected with HIV, you need to look to other components within the causal chain resulting in AIDS to prevent their condition worsening. These components include issues like adequacy of nutrition and the immune system, failures in which cannot cause progression to AIDS (not sufficient causes), but do contribute to the risk of developing AIDS. While what represents an adequate immune system is likely to be similar for everyone, adequacy of nutrition varies with age, gender, occupation, living environment, and so on. The causal chain becomes much more complicated and identifying how to intervene more challenging. While understanding the notion of necessary and sufficient causes is helpful, it is often difficult to identify the necessity and sufficiency of many causes of health and social problems.

Causal pathways

We often talk about **determinants** or **risk factors** rather than causes because of the complex causal pathways behind many outcomes and the methodological rigour around establishing that a relationship is causal. A risk factor or determinant (they are used interchangeably) is a variable associated with an increased risk of an outcome. For example, there is no single cause of obesity, but there are many risk factors including the availability of high-calorie foods, genetic factors, poverty and food access. A population group with high levels of obesity is likely to have multiple risk factors.

Thinking again of HIV infection, there are a number of ways that someone can become infected, including unprotected sex, sharing needles or transmission from mother to child during pregnancy. We call these the **proximal** or downstream causes. Proximal means close to in time or space. If we next think about what might cause those incidents that led to infection, they could include the inaccessibility of contraceptives, or inadequate control of the mother's HIV. The more proximal a factor is, the shorter the causal pathway is to the problem. If you develop an intervention that addresses these more proximal factors, then it will be easier to attribute the influence of the intervention to that problem. However, it does not mean that it is the most important causal factor. For example, lack of knowledge of healthy eating is a proximal factor for an unhealthy diet, but access to healthy foods is probably much more important.

Further upstream are policies and practices related to drug users where a needle exchange scheme or safe houses for injecting might help, and further again are issues like culture and beliefs around sex. These are called **distal** or upstream causes. A distal cause is more distant or further away in time or place than its effect. Distal causes can have amplifying affects (that is, affect some of the more proximal factors) and as such can be a highly effective target for an intervention.

This illustrates the point often made when talking about public health: we are looking for the causes of the causes. Providing a person with condoms might prevent one new infection, whereas altering policies around intravenous drug use or contraceptive supply could prevent multiple cases. While intervening on a proximal cause is likely to address that specific problem, distal cause interventions have the potential to address the breadth of problems related to that upstream cause. Within the COVID-19 pandemic, face masks and social distancing reduced transmission of the virus (proximal factors), while policies around how animals are kept might have reduced the emergence of the virus in the first place (distal factors).

Some argue that this distinction between upstream and downstream is not helpful for the development of interventions as studies have demonstrated the interaction of causes at multiple levels within systems relevant to population health (Sniehotta et al., 2017). Sniehotta and colleagues suggest that what is more important is to look at the interaction of multiple levels within systems relevant to population health. We cover the importance of systems in subsequent sections of this chapter.

Relevance of causality to intervention development

Understanding causality (or, in the case of complex problems, the risk factors and determinants) is essential to the development of interventions, and how to identify them is discussed in more detail later. Briefly, you need to understand the following points.

Knowledge link:
This topic is
also covered in
Chapter 4

The number and contribution of the risk factors to the problem you wish to address

As mentioned previously, social problems such as low education attainment, female disempowerment and alcohol misuse have multiple and complex determinants. They may range from the individual (lack of knowledge) to structural (gender bias) levels. It is often not within your power or control to change structural determinants, but you need to understand the whole range of factors in order to have a realistic idea of the effect an intervention may have. Giving someone a leaflet on healthy eating will only have marginal impact on eating patterns because the overall contribution of lack of knowledge to the problem of obesity is usually small. Compare it to the much larger contribution of the obesogenic environment (our transition to more sedentary lifestyles, the development of processed foods and access to affordable healthy foods).

Their position in the causal pathway (i.e. whether they are proximal or distal?)

Intervening upon proximal and downstream causes is common as these causes (eating sugary foods) can be quite specific in terms of the outcome they cause (dental caries), and therefore it is easier to prove the causal relationship and demonstrate the effectiveness of an intervention. Focusing on intervening on upstream causes may result in changing multiple outcomes (reducing poverty may increase individuals' ability to buy healthier

Knowledge link:
This topic is
also covered in
Chapter 2

foods and to live in better homes) but the causal relationship is more difficult to prove. However, if it is possible to intervene on an upstream cause there is the potential to reduce many outcomes.

Relevance of causality to intervention evaluation

Knowledge link:
This topic is
also covered in
Chapter 9

The Bradford Hill criteria are quite an extensive list, so how do we go about demonstrating a causal relationship in the field of human health? As an illustration, we are going to use a fictional example, shown in Figure 3.1, of an injection designed to prevent spots/acne which also seems to cause some people's hair to go grey. For illustrative purposes, we have deliberately not used a complex social problem! For a more comprehensive discussion of this matter, see Chapter 9. The four issues to consider when determining whether the change in hair colour was caused by the injection are listed in the figure and discussed below.

You have developed a new injection to prevent people getting spots/acne. You have conducted trials of the injection in the laboratory and are now ready to test the injection on humans.

Stage 1: Before and after study. You recruit 16 teenagers, give them the injection and ask them to keep a diary of how many spots they get over the next fortnight.

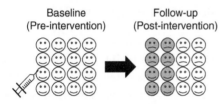

The hair of eight of the 16 teenagers turned grey, some of whom developed spots and some did not. So, what might you try next to see if the injection might have caused the grey hair?

Stage 2: Adding a *control* group. These allow you to compare what happens in the presence and absence of the intervention.

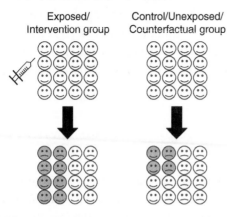

Four of the people in the control group also had their hair turn grey, so we are less certain that the injection caused the grey hair.
1. What if it was something else that you did that caused some people's hair to go grey? (*Hawthorn/observer and placebo effects*)
2. What if the four people in the control group whose hair went grey managed to get the injection elsewhere? (*Contamination*)
3. What if there were more people who were going to get grey hair in the intervention group than the control group? (*Randomisation or Matching*)

Figure 3.1 Did the injection cause people's hair to go grey?

Control groups

If you only study people who are exposed to the potential cause, you cannot tell if the outcome results from that cause or not.

Solution

Whenever possible, you want a control group to help you understand how the outcome might change in the absence of the potential cause. It might seem odd to spend money collecting data from people who have not been exposed to the potential cause, but having a control group makes a huge difference to your ability to attribute the change in an outcome to a cause or an intervention. Without a control group, none of the remaining three points can be taken into consideration. This is where the 'controlled' in a **randomised controlled trial** comes from and that is why randomised controlled trials are often described as the gold standard for effectiveness research. In other evaluation designs such as natural experiments, the control group might be called a counterfactual or an unexposed group.

Hawthorne/observer and placebo effects

There is the potential that something you did as part of the study, other than administering the injection, caused participants' hair to go grey. What if part of the recruitment process includes giving people a shock which causes some people's hair to go grey? There are two named effects to consider here: the placebo effect and the Hawthorne/observer effect. The placebo effect is the phenomenon whereby someone responds to an ineffective treatment. While it is no longer considered ethical to offer people in a medical trial a treatment which we know does not work, some people will still respond to a treatment which should not have an effect. The Hawthorne/observer effect was proposed following a trial in an office where they changed the environment (lighting and shift structure) to try to improve productivity, but even those whose office environment did not change showed an improvement in productivity. The researchers proposed that the control group also increased their productivity as they were being observed and were more aware of the need to be productive. Imagine an intervention to improve diet, and as part of the baseline data collection for the study you ask people about what they eat. It might be possible that this data collection makes people reflect on their diet so they change it, even if they don't receive the intervention. This is an example of the Hawthorne/observer effect. There is now debate about whether the Hawthorne/observer effect existed in the study that inspired it, but it is useful to think about whether any of your evaluation procedures might inappropriately influence what you find.

Solution

To address this problem, you need to try to ensure that the treatment of the exposed/ intervention and control groups are as similar as possible, apart from the potential cause or intervention. This means collecting the same data using the same techniques from both groups. This might not be enough, so we often talk about 'blinding' within an evaluation. If you blind the participants within a drug trial, each participant does not know which treatment they are receiving, so their behaviour is less likely to be affected. You could also blind the people working with the participants, so they won't treat them differently. Finally, you can also blind the person analysing the data so they don't intentionally or unintentionally bias the analysis. It is important to note that it is often challenging to blind participants in social research, compared with drug trials.

Contamination

Humans are fantastically resourceful and unpredictable, so might manage to be exposed to the potential cause even if you did not intend them to be. The four people in the control group might have heard about the new injection and managed to get it from another source to prevent their spots/acne. This is unlikely to happen when the potential cause is highly controlled, like access to pharmaceuticals. But, imagine the potential cause was an ingredient in a new product available in the supermarket. If the product is being advertised, maybe people in the control group tried it anyway?

Preventing contamination

The most common approach taken to prevent contamination is to put some distance between the exposed and control groups – so, using two wards in different hospitals, or two different schools under different education authorities. This can be important for the evaluation of your intervention. If you piloted your intervention, you want to make sure that no one who participated in the pilot ends up in the control group, which can mean recruiting in new areas for your evaluation.

Randomisation and matching

You might just have been unfortunate and ended up with four people in the control group and eight people in the exposed group whose hair was going to go grey during the study, regardless of whether they receive the injection or not. What if there had been more women in one group than the other and the outcome was more common in women, or more older people and the outcome was age related?

Solution

The first potential solution is to match people in the exposed and control groups. So, if you recruit a 30-year-old male to the exposed group, you match them with a 30-year-old male in the control group. You can match on lots of characteristics such as age, gender, socioeconomic status, ethnicity, occupation or health. Your intention is to try to match on characteristics which might alter the likelihood of the outcome, so the work you do in Step 1 of 6SQuID on the causes of the problem you are intervening to prevent is helpful. However, it is likely that there are a lot of factors which cause the problem on which you might want to match. This would be really complicated, and it is possible that you might not easily be able to observe some of the factors on which you want to match. Imagine that you want to match on the existing level of risk for a disease: you are unlikely to be able to do this without significant medical investigations. One approach to address this is called **propensity score matching**, where you use the observable matching factors within a statistical logistic regression model to find people who have similar propensity to be exposed to the potential cause, but only give one of them the potential cause or only one of them actually is exposed. The use of the propensity scores is intended to account for observed and unobservable factors in the matching, but this does not always seem to work. The optimal solution to this problem is randomisation, allocating people to the exposed/intervention or control groups randomly using random numbers, a coin toss or other random process. The problem is addressed, as random assignment means that any differences between the control and exposed groups at baseline are due to chance. Therefore, if you treat both groups the same, apart from the potential cause, any differences between the exposed/intervention and control groups at the end of the study can be attributed to the potential cause.

Knowledge link:
This topic is also covered in
Chapter 4

This fictitious example has illustrated how causality is often operationalised in evaluation research. The most common method for studying causal relationships in health research is the randomised controlled trial. However, this method is best suited to simple or complicated interventions, not complex interventions like the ones we discuss in this book.

Knowledge link:
This topic is also covered in
Chapter 4

As you can see, causality is a complicated topic. For example, you can have reciprocal causation, particularly around the relationship between humans and the environment. In order to make motor vehicle travel easier, we built more roads, which means homes can be built further from amenities, which makes active travel (e.g. walking or cycling) more difficult, which means people drive more and we need more roads. Each causal relationship in that example seems fairly logical and linear, but together we can see the system which is feeding back on itself. So, what is the specific cause, and when can you intervene? There are systems involved in the causal chain in the example and, consequently, it is important to recognise the properties of systems and their impacts on intervention development and evaluation.

SYSTEMS AND COMPLEXITY

A system can be described as 'a set of actors, activities and settings that are directly or indirectly perceived to have influence in or be affected by a given problem situation' (Foster-Fishman et al., 2007: 198). The concept of systems can be demonstrated by examples of ecosystems many of us learnt about in school. Ecosystems involve animals, plants and environments interacting together and producing constant changes, but most of the time the ecosystem remains stable.

Complexity is 'a scientific theory which asserts that some systems display behavioural phenomena that are completely inexplicable by any conventional analysis of the systems' constituent parts' (Hawe et al., 2004: 1561). In other words, a complex system is one that is adaptive to changes in its local environment, is composed of other complex systems (think of the systems in the human body) and behaves in a non-linear fashion (i.e. the change in outcome is not proportional to the change in input). A systems approach includes consideration of both indirect as well direct impacts of interventions; the contexts within which they are implemented; the relations between the multiple factors at play; and ways in which systems adapt in response to change. Complex systems are defined by several properties, including emergence, feedback and adaptation. Each of these will be considered in turn.

Emergence

Emergence refers to the properties of a complex system that cannot be directly predicted from the elements within it and are more than just the sum of its parts. For example, the changing distribution of obesity across the population can be conceptualised as an emergent property of the food, employment, transport, economic and other systems that shape the energy intake and expenditure of individuals. Stability is also an **emergent property** of the system – the individual animals, plants and environments are actively involved in this stability – it is the result of the interactions between the animals, plants and environments. Only changes like an overpopulation of one of the animals, or a plant dying out, will cause major changes in the ecosystem; sometimes these can be catastrophic, causing the whole ecosystem to collapse. We recognise that these major changes in the ecosystem are often caused by external influences, such as humans cutting down trees or overusing chemicals in farming. So, while it is easier to think about an ecosystem on its own, it is actually linked to multiple other systems.

Feedback loops

Feedback describes the situation in which a change may reinforce or balance further change. For example, the relationship between diet and disease can be a cycle where diseases such as cholera can lead to poor nutritional status, and ultimately malnutrition. These then become risk factors for other diseases. A poorly nourished adult or child is more likely to develop disease; an ill person may need more or fewer calories or absorb calories less efficiently. Although both inadequate dietary intake and disease can independently contribute to conditions such as malnutrition, it is often a result of the combination of both the disease and the risk factor. Figure 3.2 demonstrates a causal loop diagram illustrating some of the interacting components in a society responding to the threat of COVID-19. A reinforcing feedback loop is responsible for causing exponential growth in the number of infected people. However, the risk of transmission is seen to be a factor of the context and the systems in place, not simply a characteristic of the virus. As such, there are many dynamic interactions involving components such as the public's trust in authorities. The example of building roads is a positive or reinforcing feedback loop, where more roads lead to more roads. Often in nature, we find negative or balancing feedback loops; for example, when the level of sugar in our blood rises, a negative feedback loop happens to reduce the level of sugar by removing it from the blood stream to be used by the tissues or stored for use later. However, when humans become involved, systems become more complicated and even complex.

The causes of any outcome or behaviour are often embedded in the systems in which that outcome or behaviour occurs. In the example of Kieran's headaches, we learned that the practices and culture at his workplace have been contributing to his headaches. In order to prevent his headaches, it was necessary for Kieran to involve his line manager and workplace to make changes that were out of his control. These changes might have implications for the businesses Kieran's employer works with as they are all linked together in a system, potentially preventing headaches for employees of those other businesses. Grant and Hood (2017) illustrated the systems around a 'sugar tax' on soft drinks that need to be understood to evaluate whether the tax was successful. They give the example that, as supermarkets are under pressure to maintain sales, they might introduce special offers to reduce the costs and maintain sales, so you might not observe a reduction in sales as you hoped. Whenever your intervention is intended to alter human behaviour, it is likely that there will be multiple systems that need to be considered. Intervening without consideration of these systems can have unexpected and/or harmful consequences.

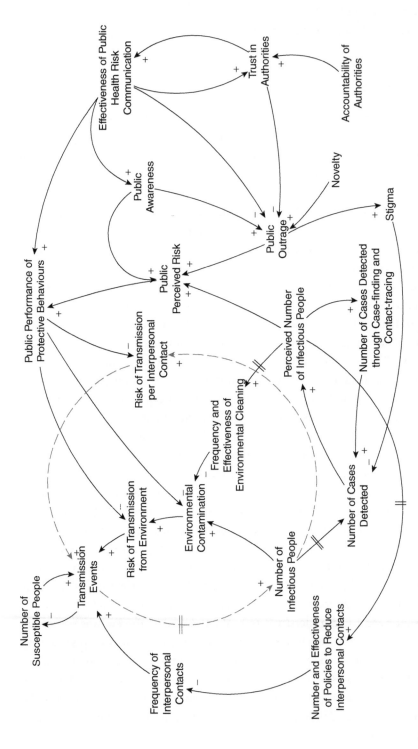

Figure 3.2 An example causal loop diagram illustrating some of the interacting components in a society responding to the threat of COVID-19

Reproduced by kind permission of Elsevier ltd

Source: Bradley et al. (2020)

Systems interact with other systems, individual parts of one system might leave one system and join another, and the behaviour of one system might influence one or more other systems. Often, the interactions within a system can cause feedback loops like the example of reciprocal causation given above.

Adaptation

Adaptation refers to adjustments in behaviour in response to interventions or changes made. A complex approach helps to understand the wider implications of the intervention and the interactions that occur between components of interventions. To illustrate that a complex system can adapt in order to survive with the removal of one of its parts, we could think of a prison system. The removal of a single warden will not destroy the system as other prison wardens can compensate for the loss. Moreover, the addition of one more warden will not significantly make the system more efficient, i.e. there is no dose–response relationship. Grant and Hood (2017), in their example of a sugar tax on soft drinks, describe how the complex system of retail might adapt to a simple intervention like a new tax on sugary products. Careful consideration of the systems around an intervention like a sugar tax can help to ensure that the intervention is successful, by identifying and mitigating for any changes in the system that might reduce the intervention effect.

Activity 3.1

Why did I have toast for breakfast?

Try thinking about why you ate whatever you ate for breakfast this morning. Start with your individual choices/behaviours, why you might or might not have had breakfast, and whether you prefer toast, cereal or something else. What social and cultural factors might be informing your breakfast choice? Then think about the practical issues: what if you didn't have what you wanted for breakfast in the cupboard, or did not have equipment to make your breakfast, like a toaster? Think about where the ingredients in your breakfast came from, how the electricity was generated so you could boil the kettle, if it was possible to have what you really wanted or whether it was available in your local shop. Why did you want to eat when you woke up? Why did you wake up at that time? Even a fairly simply behaviour like having breakfast is part of multiple systems. Changes in any one of those systems might alter the outcome (what you had for breakfast).

SIMPLE, COMPLICATED AND COMPLEX INTERVENTIONS

An intervention exerts its influence by changing relationships, displacing existing activities and redistributing and transforming resources (Hawe et al., 2009). An intervention can be remedial, seeking to reduce a problem once it has occurred, sometimes called treatment or curative. Or an intervention can be preventive, seeking to prevent a problem before it occurs. With either a remedial or preventive social intervention, we often classify interventions as simple, complicated or complex in relation to the attributes of the causal factors, and how they interact with the systems involved. In the context of this book, interventions aimed at reducing social determinants of health are almost always complex. Rogers (2008) suggests that simple and complicated interventions should address aspects of the agencies (single and multi) involved in implementation; and whether the interventions have multiple and/or alternative causal strands. Alternative causal strand/linear causality suggests that different causal mechanisms may be operating in different contexts. It is important to understand the relative strength of each causal strand in order to have the best mix of intervention components. While it is possible to pre-identify outcomes, whether these are achieved may be dependent on factors such as the training of staff and the consistency of delivery (intervention fidelity). Unexpected effects seen when interventions are implemented can sometimes relate to the complexity of the systems in which the intervention is introduced. Recognition of the complexity of systems began in the field of physics and has now been applied across the sciences as we recognise more aspects of life as complex adaptive systems. We have described the characteristics of complex adaptive systems above, and now consider what they mean when developing and evaluating interventions.

Simple interventions

A simple intervention can be defined as a standardised intervention with a single causal strand that links the intervention and its outcome. Many drug interventions, screening and immunisation programmes could be described as simple interventions. The properties of a simple intervention are listed below, and Table 3.1 provides examples of each property:

- a linear, single causal pathway which could imply that the system can be decomposed into its parts, where each part solves separate problems in order to have a complete answer
- focused on one main cause
- dose–response, whereby more of the intervention causes more effect
- fairly straightforward to replicate
- outcomes that can be pre-identified
- often implemented by a single governing organisation.

CAUSALITY, SYSTEMS AND COMPLEXITY **51**

Table 3.1 Simple intervention example: Use of vaccination against poliomyelitis

Simplicity criteria	Description	Further description
Single causal strand	Poliomyelitis is only caused by poliovirus – it is a necessary cause (assuming you have the necessary viral load to develop the disease). There is a direct linear relationship between the poliovirus and getting poliomyelitis	Universal causal mechanism regardless of population or location
Intervention works through one main causal and linear path	The polio vaccine (intervention) acts on poliovirus (causal strand) to prevent poliomyelitis (outcome)	The same vaccination can be used in different countries on the same population group without modification
Dose – response relationship – so the more effort invested, the greater the reward	Population approaches to vaccination are most effective – ad hoc vaccination of individuals may not be cost-effective and high uptake is important	Mass vaccination programmes
Single agency	The health department in a community/state is usually responsible for vaccination governance and training	The effectiveness of the intervention is not affected by the person delivering the intervention. There are standardised protocols and training
Highly replicable intervention	The vaccination is standardised and regulated. There are standardised training and procedures for storing and delivering the vaccination	Once the training has been undertaken, the attributes of the person delivering the vaccine should be irrelevant and not affect delivery. The intervention's effectiveness is not dependent on the person delivering the intervention
Outcomes can be pre-identified	Very high certainty that vaccination will prevent poliomyelitis in an individual	The outcome has a high degree of certainty and is easy to measure

Complicated interventions

Complicated interventions are those with many components (because the health 'problem' has multiple causal strands) which operate in different contexts and so do not necessarily interact but produce a common outcome. The properties of complicated interventions are listed below, and Table 3.2 provides examples of each property:

- the intervention can work either through one or other causal pathways
- the causal pathways are linear, often implying that the system can be decomposed into its parts, where each part solves separate problems in order to have a complete solution
- dose–response, whereby more of the intervention causes more effect
- can be replicated, although this might require training of those who will start delivering the intervention or creation of a manual for the intervention
- outcomes can be pre-identified
- implementation in different sites and/or under different governance.

Table 3.2 Complicated intervention example: prevention of dental caries

Aspects of the causal pathway which are complicated	Aspects of the intervention which are complicated	Further description
Multiple simultaneous causal strands. Dental caries caused by: - poor dental hygiene - poor nutrition - lack of fluoride in water	Health professionals provide education on importance of oral hygiene Schools may ban sweets and sugared beverages in lunchboxes Water companies supply fluoridated water at levels that is effective for preventing cavities	If all causal strands are relevant, an intervention may need to focus on interrupting all the causal pathways to effectively reduce dental caries
Alternative causal strand/linear causality. Some areas may have: - high levels of fluorine in water - high levels of sugar in diet - poor oral hygiene practices	if water fluoridation not necessary, focus on interventions which reduce sugar intake and increase oral hygiene	Intervention may work through several alternative strands but not all may be necessary. Need to know more about the context and strength of causal strand
Multiple agencies	Health educators, water companies, schools	Different agencies working at different levels to achieve a shared goal
Certainty of outcome	High certainty that doing the above preventative actions will prevent tooth decay	The outcome can be predicted

Complex interventions

A complex intervention is built up from a number of components, which may act both independently and inter-dependently. There are different dimensions to complexity, which may include the components of the intervention itself and the property of the systems within which the intervention operates. Complex interventions are those that are most adapted to the specific systems and contexts in which they are implemented and may be difficult to standardise, replicate and scale up. These types of interventions explicitly acknowledge that many systems are complex and adaptive. Table 3.3 lists the dimensions and characteristics of complex interventions. Rogers (2008) suggests that complex interventions should address two important features of complex systems: reciprocal or recursive causality/and disproportionate effects; and outcome emergence. An example of this is shown in Table 3.4.

These definitions of simple, complicated and complex assume that these are inherent characteristics of interventions. However, it has been argued that there may be no 'simple' or 'complex' interventions, and that '*simplicity and complexity are instead pragmatic perspectives adopted by researchers to help describe and understand the interventions in question'* (Petticrew, 2011). Our description of complex interventions makes them sound difficult. But we are very used to interacting and operating in systems. Even seemingly simple interventions like a vaccine become complex when you start to consider how the vaccine can be delivered to everyone in a population, the production and storage of the vaccine and how humans might respond to it in terms of trust in the government or science. Throughout this book, we will take you through steps in developing and evaluating interventions within complex systems, whether the intervention ends up being simple, complicated or complex.

Table 3.3 Dimensions and properties of complex interventions

Dimensions of complexity (Craig et al., 2011: 7)	Characteristics of complex interventions (Pawson and Tilley, 2004)
• Number of and interactions between components within the experimental and control interventions • Number and difficulty of behaviours required by those delivering or receiving the intervention • Number of groups or organisational levels targeted by the intervention • Number and variability of outcomes • Degree of flexibility or tailoring of the intervention permitted	• Have an underlying theory or theories • Involve the actions of people • Consist of a chain of steps or processes • These chains of steps or processes are often not linear • Are embedded in social systems • Are prone to modification • Are open systems which change through learning

Table 3.4 Complex intervention example: alcohol brief interventions (ABI)

Complexity criteria and background	Aspects of complex interventions	Further description
Recursive causality and disproportionate effect - A positive experience of not drinking helps the person envisage not drinking in other environments in a positive feedback loop - The ABI is enough of a trigger to help someone give up drinking, while for another it has no effect	Various components of the brief interventions interact with each other to produce different drinking outcome patterns. So, it is difficult to tell which aspects will have the most impact on drinking behaviour	Input and output not directly correlated. The motivational interviewing skills, person delivering the ABI, timing of the intervention, and motivations of the client may all be important
Emergence/evolving outcome	Brief intervention could lead to reduction in alcohol consumption or abstinence or there will be no effect. May affect other outcomes such as domestic violence, smoking habits	Uncertainties as to how a person will respond to the intervention. The ABI may not be the reason people stop drinking or the intervention might lead to a change in the local culture and to much broader unintended effects

---

Activity 3.2

Simple, complicated or complex?

Consider the following three interventions:

- Adding a pedestrian crossing to a road
- Installing a stair gate when your child starts walking
- Organising a party

For each intervention:

1. Identity whether the interventions could be described as simple, complicated or complex.
2. Describe the aspects that make them simple, complicated or complex.
3. Think about the implications of the intervention type on how the intervention would be developed.

CAUSAL FACTORS, SYSTEMS AND COMPLEXITY IN INTERVENTION DEVELOPMENT

Having recognised the causal factors, systems and complexity related to your intervention, what does this mean for developing and delivering interventions? There are cross-cutting factors that influence, interact and impact one in many systems such as healthcare, transport and education. These may include:

- policies and governance;
- financing and budgets;
- information and communications;
- infrastructure, resources and supplies;
- service delivery and production; and
- the sociocultural environment.

Think about implementing physical activity classes in a workplace and which of the above you may need to negotiate or take into account before you start delivery. You may need to know what health and safety policies are in place; whether there is a budget for equipment, or a room to hold the class; how the workforce will know the classes are taking place; how the classes fit in with work breaks and expectations of productivity; and finally whether anyone will turn up or there is a culture of sitting at one's desk for lunch. Anticipating these in advance, and developing interventions to take account of them, will greatly increase the chances of success.

Another issue when intervening in complex systems is that of what to do in relation to reciprocal/recursive causality, or the outcomes that are emergent and unpredictable. There are no easy answers to these questions and many academics debate this topic.

However, we would like to present two useful ideas that have been proposed around causation in complex systems.

The first idea is to think about the contribution to an outcome of a component of an intervention in a system (Forss et al., 2011). This recognises that full understanding of the causes of an outcome is difficult, but we might be able to understand how a specific cause contributes to the problem. Contribution analysis has been developed to examine the contribution of interventions and systems (Mayne, 2011). The second idea proposed by Rod et al. (2014) talks about the spirit of an intervention out of recognition that, however well an intervention may be designed, once it starts to be implemented it is adapted and shaped by the systems around it. If you maintain the spirit of the intervention, but do not deliver it exactly as described on paper, will you achieve the same outcomes? Ideally, your intervention would allow for adaptation and we talk more about how to achieve this in Chapters 6 and 7.

Knowledge link: This topic is also covered in Chapters 6 and 7

Activity 3.3

Masks and COVID-19

The novel nature of COVID-19 meant that a simple intervention like face masks was introduced to control the spread of the infection, until other control methods like a vaccination were developed. Although masks seem like a simple intervention, can you write down some of the systems related to this intervention? Think about both practical (e.g. manufacture and distribution) and psychological (e.g. attitudes and anxieties) aspects of the intervention.

SUMMARY

In this chapter, we have introduced the concepts of causality, systems and complexity. A thorough understanding of causality, systems and complexity have implications for the whole process of developing and evaluating an intervention. Systems and complexity are part of our everyday lives, from the systems within the cells of our bodies, up to international financial systems and solar systems. By recognising and describing causal factors, areas of complexity and the systems which impact on your problem, you should be able to take account of them (to some extent) in the development of your intervention. This complexity might create challenges in the development and evaluation of the intervention. However, by incorporating an understanding of systems into the development of your intervention, it is more likely to be sustainable and effective.

FURTHER READING

Forss, K., Marra, M., and Schwartz, R. (2011) *Evaluating the Complex: Attribution, Contribution, and Beyond*. Abingdon: Transaction Publishers.

Hawe, P., Shiell, A., and Riley, T. (2009) 'Theorising interventions as events in systems', *American Journal of Community Psychology*, 43 (3–4): 267–76.

REFERENCES

Bradley, D., Mansouri, M., Kee, F., and Garcia, L. (2020) 'A systems approach to preventing and responding to COVID-19', *EClinicalMedicine, 21*: 100325.

Craig, P., Cooper, C., Gunnell, D., Haw, S., Lawson, K., Macintyre, S., Ogilvie, D., Petticrew, M., Reeves, B., Sutton, M., and Thompson, S. (2011) *Using Natural Experiments to Evaluate Population Health Interventions: Guidance for Producers and Users of Evidence.* London: Medical Research Council. www.mrc.ac.uk/documents/pdf/natural-experiments-guidance, accessed 11 June 2020.

Forss, K., Marra, M., and Schwartz, R. (2011) *Evaluating the Complex: Attribution, Contribution, and Beyond.* Abingdon: Transaction Publishers.

Foster-Fishman, P. G., Nowell, B., and Yang, H. (2007) 'Putting the system back into systems change: a framework for understanding and changing organizational and community systems', *American Journal of Community Psychology, 39* (3–4): 197–215.

Grant, R. L., and Hood, R. (2017) 'Complex systems, explanation and policy: implications of the crisis of replication for public health research', *Critical Public Health, 27* (5): 525–32.

Hawe, P., Shiell, A., and Riley, T. (2004) 'Complex interventions: how "out of control" can a randomised controlled trial be?', *BMJ, 328* (7455): 1561–3.

Hawe, P., Shiell, A., and Riley, T. (2009) 'Theorising interventions as events in systems', *American Journal of Community Psychology, 43* (3–4): 267–76.

Hill, A. B. (1965) 'The environment and disease: association or causation?', *Proceedings of the Royal Society of Medicine, 58*: 295–300.

Mayne, J. (2011) 'Contribution analysis: addressing cause and effect', in K. Forss, M. Marra and R. Schwartz (eds), *Evaluating the Complex: Attribution, Contribution and Beyond.* Abingdon: Transaction Publishers, pp. 53–96.

Parascandola, M., and Weed, D. L. (2001) 'Causation in epidemiology', *Journal of Epidemiology and Community Health, 55* (12): 905–12.

Pawson, R. and Tilley, N. (2004) *Realist Evaluation.* London: Sage Publications.

Petticrew, M. (2011) 'When are complex interventions "complex"? When are simple interventions "simple"?', *European Journal of Public Health, 21* (4): 397–8.

Rod, M. H., Ingholt, L., Sorensen, B. B., and Tjornhoj-Thomsen, T. (2014) 'The spirit of the intervention: reflections on social effectiveness in public health intervention research', *Critical Public Health, 24* (3): 296–307.

Rogers, P. J. (2008) 'Using programme theory to evaluate complicated and complex aspects of interventions', *Evaluation, 14*: 29–48.

Sniehotta, F. F., Araujo-Soares, V., Brown, J., Kelly, M. P., Michie, S., and West, R. (2017) 'Complex systems and individual-level approaches to population health: a false dichotomy?', *The Lancet Public Health, 2* (9): e396–e397.

ACTIVITY ANSWERS

Activity 3.1: Why did I have toast for breakfast?

Individual factors

- You might have woken up late and had to skip breakfast
- You forgot to buy bread so cannot have the toast you would usually have

- The toaster was broken
- You need some nutrition to prepare you for the day

Social and cultural factors

- Your peers do not have breakfast so neither do you
- All the popular people are having avocado toast, so you try to have that as well
- It has become a tradition in your family to have porridge for breakfast
- Your religious beliefs mean that you do not eat meat, so you do not have a full English breakfast

Structural factors

- There is a power cut/outage so you have to get breakfast on the way to work
- The weather produced a poor wheat crop last year so you cannot have bread for breakfast
- The company that makes the cereal you like has increased their prices, so you have switched to something else.

Activity 3.2: Simple, complicated or complex?

1. Adding a pedestrian crossing to a road, despite sounding fairly simple, is an example of a complex intervention. You need to understand and adapt the intervention around the street and road use systems. There is no point in putting a crossing where no one is walking, and if you put the crossing just after some traffic lights you might cause lots of congestion. If you put it close to a junction, it might be difficult for drivers to notice it early and take appropriate action. The implications of this are:

    a. A strong theoretical understanding of how the intervention changes the systems around it is necessary to identify and strengthen weak components in the causal chain.
    b. Specific outcome measures may be difficult to identify in advance. The new crossing might cause people to start taking that route and increase business in the area. Drivers might not notice the new crossing, causing an increase in collisions and casualties. You might divert people from another crossing, making that crossing pointless.
    c. You will have to collect data on a wide variety of outcomes to try to detect the impact of the intervention.
    d. Lack of increases in people walking may not mean the intervention is ineffective but may be due to implementation issues, like it being in the wrong place.
    e. Complexities within these systems mean that it would be best to work with local organisations and communities to identify where the crossing should be placed.

2. Installing a stair gate when your child starts walking is an example of a simple intervention. You are trying to prevent your child getting hurt by falling down the stairs, so you place

the gate at the top of the stairs. In the long run, you will help your child develop the skills and dexterity to both recognise stairs and be able to use them safely, but that takes more time and is more complex. The simple intervention can give you time to intervene in the more complex system. The implications of this intervention are that it is fairly easy to replicate and evaluate as the causal chain is linear. There could be other intervention options to intervene in this causal chain, like having people live on one floor when they have a young child, or not allowing the child to move around more freely, but obviously these are more difficult interventions and less acceptable.

3. Organising a party is an example of a complicated intervention. There are multiple aspects to the party, like who to invite, where to hold it, the food, the music. These are all important for making the party successful, but maybe you could have the party in a different place, or with different food, and still have a good party. Knowing all the components of the party, you can plan and manage each aspect (identifying a caterer, deciding what food to have, managing its delivery, etc.). Here are some implications of a complicated intervention:

    a. They can pose a challenge to evaluation, due to many components. People might tell you that the party was good, but they did not like the music. Does that make it a bad party?

    b. An intervention with many causal strands must focus on all components simultaneously, but where resources are scarce there could be an assessment to identify the most potent causal strands. Maybe if your budget is tight, your friends will not mind if you just have a playlist for the music rather than live music, but if your friends are classical music enthusiasts, this might completely ruin the party.

    c. Because of its many causal strands, it is difficult for evaluation to properly identify and investigate all the components. Later on, you want a similar party, but in a different location, and you don't know from the original party whether the location helped make it successful or did not really matter.

    d. But when you have developed your formula for the perfect party, it becomes easier to replicate as there is a high degree of certainty of outcome.

Activity 3.3: Masks and COVID-19

1. Manufacturers' systems and their suppliers – needed to create the masks
2. Distribution and transport systems – to get the masks to where they are needed for sale
3. Marketing and selling of the masks – to get the masks to the population
4. Cultural systems including community and family – to create norms around mask wearing
5. Public health and health promotion – to make people aware of the importance of wearing masks
6. Media – to increase awareness and may reinforce cultural norms

4
6SQuID STEP 1: UNDERSTANDING THE PROBLEM AND ITS CAUSES

Learning objectives

After reading this chapter, you will be able to:

- Understand how to choose and define a problem
- Carry out a problem analysis with your intervention development team (your stake-holders) to determine the root causes
- Visually represent the problem.

Scenario 4.1

A community gambling problem

Jendyose has been thinking about a problem that has been brought to her attention in her role as Director of Public Health in a rural area of Uganda. Since the turn of the century, the gambling industry in Uganda has increased rapidly, with various new facilities being intro-duced. The proliferation of gambling has seen the industry diversify from casino gambling

(Continued)

and national lotteries to new modes like sports betting and online betting. Members of her local community are worried about the effect that gambling is having on families. Some are struggling to feed their children as they run up huge debts. The community is trying to support them but the problem seems to be getting worse. Jendyose needs to understand the causes of the community gambling problem by asking appropriate questions. This process is called problem analysis. What sort of questions might she ask?

INTRODUCTION

The first step of developing an intervention is to understand the problem you are hoping to address. Once you have clearly defined the problem, you can start to understand the contributory factors and systems at play. This process will increase the likelihood that you arrive at the right conclusions in relation to how to address the problem, which will then increase the likelihood of your programme's success.

This chapter will describe how to fully articulate the problem an intervention (or programme) is trying to address, including:

- Deciding on the problem to address;
- Defining the problem;
- Determining the causes of the problem and the systems in which it exists;
- Describing what interventions have been tried before to address the problem (and why they did or did not work).

DECIDING ON THE PROBLEM TO ADDRESS

The 6SQuID framework begins with the premise that a problem has already been identified. Sometimes, this step will have been undertaken for you by grant funders; governments (with priorities such as the United Nations' Sustainable Development Goals); supervisors; or local public health decision makers. For example, many grant funders will ask researchers to formulate a research project around a specific topic area, or public health policy makers will have undertaken a prioritisation exercise. Occasionally, an issue like COVID-19 will emerge as the dominant problem that needs urgent solutions. However, you could also identify a topic area based upon your personal and professional experiences or the issues your community has raised. Problems identified by existing research can also guide problem selection.

If you have not already identified a problem or a need and are working in a local community or area, you may want to undertake a **needs assessment**. A need is an important concept in public health, with no universal definition. Bradshaw (1972) identified four types of need – normative need, felt need, expressed need and comparative need. A normative need is a need identified according to a norm or standard. This norm may be defined by an expert such as the vaccination identified by experts as a solution to control the spread of COVID-19. A felt need is a need perceived by an individual. Felt needs are often constrained by individual knowledge and perceptions of services. For example, an individual with diabetes might feel that there should be a diabetes clinic in the community. A felt need that has been turned into an action is called an expressed need. For instance, an individual who feels that a diabetes clinic is needed in a community takes an action by mobilising the community and resources to set up a diabetes clinic. Comparative need is a need identified by comparing the service received by one group with those received by another group. For example, a village may notice that there is a mental health facility in a neighbouring village which provides great support to the people of that village and this may influence their need to establish a similar facility in their own village.

Needs assessments help to identify and understand needs or problems to address that are specific to your local area. The section below will briefly describe how to conduct a needs assessment, prior to beginning Step 1 of 6SQuID. (For a more thorough step-by-step approach to needs assessment, see Green and Kreuter (2005)). Needs assessments not only cover health needs and behaviours but also assess the external or environmental factors leading to the problem. For example, a needs assessment of gambling behaviours in Scotland found that young men felt 'bombarded' by marketing campaigns in their everyday lives, whereas women and older men felt better able to resist these. These types of risk factors (for gambling) can influence who the problem affects most and which population an intervention should target.

A needs assessment usually entails a full description of the problem, a preliminary understanding of the causes, as well as the perspective of stakeholders such as those affected by or concerned about the problem. This contextualises the problem and maximises the chances that any subsequently developed intervention will address the needs of those impacted by the problem. A needs assessment should be approached systematically to fully understand the needs of the community or population. One method suggested by Green and Kreuter (2005) is to develop a model of what is already known about the problem and what issues need to be explored further in order to obtain accurate evidence on which to base priorities and decisions. This method involves conducting a social assessment (how does the problem affect quality of life?); epidemiological assessment (how does the problem affect specific health outcomes?); and educational and ecological assessment (what knowledge, attitudes and contextual factors influence the problem?). This can clearly be quite a lengthy process in itself, but some of the activities we recommend in this chapter can help you expedite the process.

DEFINING AND UNDERSTANDING THE PROBLEM

It is critical to explicitly define and agree the problem with your team from the outset. Even if you have undertaken a needs assessment and believe you have a clear idea of the problem, you need to ensure that stakeholders feel the same way. It is easy to make the assumption that we all think about a problem in the same way, but this is not always the case. You may end up developing an intervention that is not effective because it is treating the wrong problem. This is because each of us thinks about the same problem differently because of how it affects us personally – our health, our family, our work, our resources and our policies. As a result, different stakeholders will bring different perspectives and have different needs. Consider a public health practitioner who has decided that the main problem in her community is that many children eat a poor diet. For the public health practitioner, a poor diet is one which lacks fruit and vegetables and is high in fat and sugar. However, for the single parent on a low income, a poor diet is one that does not provide enough calories to keep their child from being hungry. For the sports coach, a poor diet is one which is low in protein and does not create the muscle bulk for team competitions. All of these stakeholders need to agree and define a standard definition of 'poor diet', prior to moving forward in the intervention development process, otherwise there may be confusion and frustration about what the intervention outcomes are down the line.

The first step therefore is to understand the range of understandings of the problem and agree as a group on a definition. At the same time, you can start to think about how the problem is socially and geographically distributed.

You can use the activities below to identify issues related to distribution of the problem and its effect on health inequalities. When you have defined your problem, you want to be specific about whom the problem impacts on. You may want to consider the following questions in a workshop activity which could follow on from the defining of the problem:

- Who is impacted most by this problem?
- Where are these groups based geographically – urban or rural?
- When does the problem occur in the life course?

Explicitly defining who the problem affects can inform decisions later when considering intervention components, delivery and evaluation. Beyond the people that the problem directly impacts, think about who else may be indirectly impacted by the problem. For example, gambling by one member of the family may impact the whole family and have indirect impacts on the community and local services.

You should have already started building your 'intervention development team', made up of you and your team (if you have one) and the relevant stakeholders, so this can be one of your first tasks! A workshop format is a good way of undertaking this activity, and can be a fun and illuminating one.

INTERVENTION DEVELOPMENT TOOLS FOR DEFINING THE PROBLEM

A workshop (either online or face to face) with your intervention development team is a good way to begin the process of defining and understanding the problem. As we explained earlier, your team should consist of yourself and any colleagues (if applicable), individuals or representatives or groups who are affected by the problem, organisations representing those affected by the problem, experts, individuals who represent the different systems in which the problem is occurring, those who will be responsible for delivery of your intervention, decision makers and policy makers, and funders or those responsible for resourcing any intervention. We recognise that, in some cases, not all of the above will be applicable, for instance your team may not have received any funding. The idea here is to bring different types of knowledge and experience to the process, as much as is relevant to your circumstances, in order to increase the likelihood that your intervention will be acceptable, sustainable and effective. For workshops such as this, we would encourage you to invite other stakeholders that are not part of your immediate team but fall into any of the categories of persons previously mentioned.

Knowledge link: This topic is also covered in Chapter 2

There are several visual tools you can use in a workshop format to help your team see if they have a common understanding of the problem. Although we introduce these tools in this section, you can use them at various stages of the intervention development process.

Rich pictures

Rich pictures are a way of building a picture of the collective views and perspectives of those involved (Checkland, 2000). These are used to understand how concepts and systems link together and interact with each other. Using images and metaphors is helpful and will prompt those involved to expand their thoughts as well as providing a reminder of what the team has discussed. By building a 'rich picture' collaboratively, you will be able to see what issues and challenges emerge, as well as initial thoughts as to the inter-connectedness of these issues.

Ask your team members and wider stakeholders to draw a picture beforehand or during the workshop that describes the problem. You can also ask them to take photos to illus-trate the problem. In the scenario above about gambling, the public health practitioner might draw pictures of hungry children, and families experiencing poverty. The single parent may draw a picture of their child lying in bed crying due to hunger and the stress and anxiety they feel. Asking workshop participants to show their pictures and talk about their understandings of the problem will facilitate arrival at a common definition that all can agree on. Figure 4.1 shows a single rich picture representing how the families of the person gambling may feel in the scenario at the beginning of the chapter. The picture rep-resents their poverty, including trips to the community centre for food and clothes, and to the health centre with their sick children. There is a magnet in the centre to indicate that gamblers are drawn to various types of gambling. The industry and the government are represented as the only ones who benefit from this (via profits and taxes).

At the end of the rich pictures session, you would aim to bring all these perspec-tives together in a single picture with text, stickies, and photos added to show the links

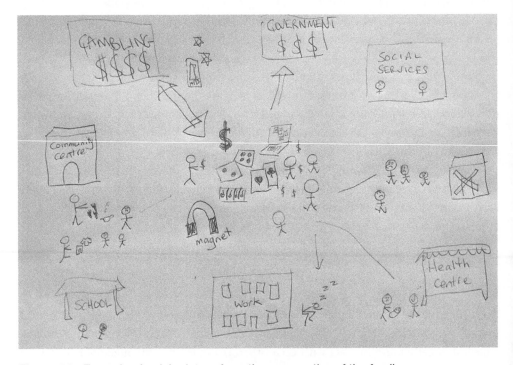

Figure 4.1   Example of a rich picture from the perspective of the family

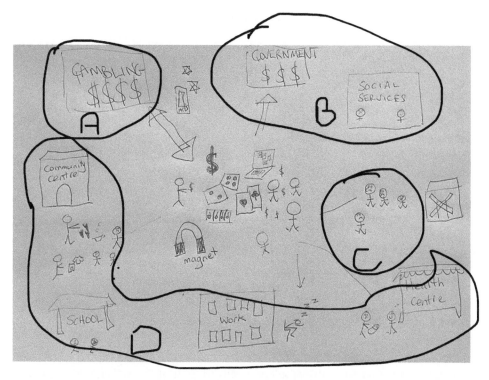

Figure 4.2 Example of a rich picture from the perspective of the family, with systems added

between institutions, physical aspects and people. You can use this approach to start to identify the different systems in which the problem occurs, as shown in Figure 4.2. In this diagram, the letter A represents industry; B represents national and local government; C represents family and community; and D represents local services and organisations. The rich pictures method is useful to identify how these systems interact.

Multi-perspective approach diagrams

A similar activity is the **multi-perspective approach** (Morgan and Ogbonna, 2008). This approach aims to capture the views of the various stakeholders in addition to what the situation means to them and what is important to them. Initially, the perspective of those present is captured, then the group imagines what the perspectives of others might be. In the example given in the scenario, we can try to imagine what gambling might mean to those involved. Figure 4.3 illustrates what Jendyose and the intervention development team might produce in relation to this task.

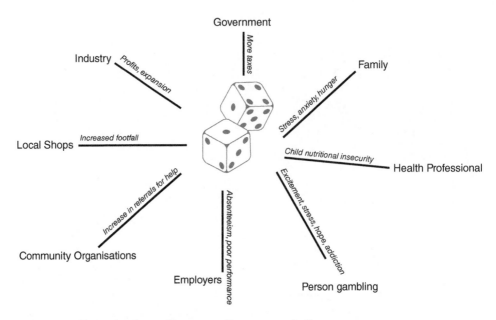

Figure 4.3   Example of a multi-perspective approach diagram

This diagram shows what the problem means to each of the stakeholders. The team then need to reach consensus as to the perspective that matters most. The ideal outcome would be to have multiple perspectives represented in the decision, but if this is not possible, then the team should think about who the problem is affecting most. Explicitly defining who the problem affects can inform decisions later when considering intervention components, delivery and evaluation. Beyond the people that the problem directly impacts, think about who else may be indirectly impacted by the issue. For example, the gambling of one member of the family may impact the whole family and have indirect impacts on the community and local services.

World Cafes

You may also wish to consider using the **World Cafe** approach, which can be done face to face or online. This approach is a simple and flexible method for hosting large group dialogue, as shown in Box 3.1 (www.theworldcafe.com). It is therefore incredibly useful for any work you might undertake that requires the input of multiple stakeholders. As the 6SQuID framework is founded upon principles of co-production, you can revisit this approach and others mentioned in this chapter as you progress through each of the steps.

CASE STUDY: COMPONENTS OF WORLD CAFES (ADAPTED FROM WWW.THEWORLDCAFE.COM)

1. Setting: Create a 'special' environment, most often modelled after a cafe, i.e. small round tables covered with a tablecloth, paper, coloured pens, a vase of flowers. There should be four chairs at each table (optimally) – and no more than five. This can be adapted for a virtual workshop by using breakout rooms. Instead of paper and pens, you can use software such as Miro (https://miro.com), IdeaBoardz (https://ideaboardz.com) or similar. The aim is to let people write or draw their thoughts, which can then be shared with others and kept as a record of discussions.
2. Welcome and Introduction: The host begins with a welcome and an introduction to the World Cafe process, setting the context, sharing the Cafe etiquette, and putting participants at ease.
3. Small-Group Rounds: The process begins with the first of three or more 20-minute rounds of conversation for small groups of four (five maximum) people seated around a table. At the end of the 20 minutes, each member of the group moves to a different table. They may or may not choose to leave one person as the 'table host' for the next round, who welcomes the next group and briefly fills them in on what happened in the previous round. In a virtual setting, a facilitator would remain in the breakout room and the participants would be moved to another breakout room.
4. Questions: Each round is prefaced with a question specially crafted for the specific context and desired purpose of the World Cafe. The same questions can be used for more than one round, or they may build upon each other to focus the conversation or guide its direction.
5. Harvest: After the small groups (and/or in between rounds, as needed), individuals are invited to share insights or other results from their conversations with the rest of the large group. These results are reflected visually in a variety of ways, most often using a visual method at the front of the room.

The World Cafe method typically involves short group conversations, with each member of the group moving to a different group after a period of time. These conversations are geared around predefined questions. Questions could focus on who is impacted most by the problem under consideration, where the problem occurs in the life course, and so on. The process culminates in what is referred to as harvesting, where the 'fruits' of the conversation are shared with the rest of the group. Ideally, results are combined visually and presented at the front of the room. Each element of the method has a specific purpose and can be modified to meet a wide variety of needs. The specifics of context, number of attendees, purpose, location, design, question choice and other circumstances are factored into each event's unique invitation.

DETERMINING THE CAUSES OF THE PROBLEM AND THE SYSTEMS INVOLVED

Knowledge link:
This topic is
also covered in
Chapter 3

We have emphasised the importance of understanding cause and effect, systems and complexity elsewhere in this book. It is necessary to have a thorough understanding of all the potential causes and how they link to systems before thinking about the intervention itself. There are many sources of data you can use to build up a picture of the range of causes and systems and their contribution to your problem. You may have already done this if you have either conducted a needs assessment, or have access to needs assessment conducted by someone else. The starting place for identifying risk factors (i.e. possible causes or determinants) is reviewing the available evidence from the scientific epidemiological literature, and also from any local epidemiological data. You will then need to share that evidence with your team to help assess it for relevance in the local context. Remember, your team should include stakeholders, and the different knowledge and experience they bring will be invaluable for contextualising any evidence you uncover. Working with your team, you should build a picture of what additional local factors are important, including the local systems which impact on the problem, since these may also impact on any intervention you develop.

Epidemiological evidence

If possible, you should try and get at least an overview of the epidemiological evidence. We recognise that this may be difficult for some, depending on the time and resources available. You can save time and resources by looking for an existing systematic review on the topic. Systematic reviews can provide rigorous overviews of what the risk factors contributing to a disease or condition are. This can be the most efficient way to understand what the contributing factors to a problem are. For example, instead of reading 60 individual studies to understand the different risk factors for asthma attacks in children, you may identify a recent systematic review that summarises the key factors across those studies.

If there are no systematic reviews, then you may need to look at individual epidemiological studies. These provide quantitative information about associations and relationships between risk factors to the cause of a problem. When looking at factors contributing to any given problem, the strongest study designs are prospective cohort studies (following a similar group of individuals over time to discover if a particular factor influences the development of an outcome) and case-control studies (studying risk factor differences in two groups: one with a relevant condition and another without). These study designs typically report correlations, i.e. relationships between two variables. They do not, however, explain that relationship – it is not possible to say that one causes the other – only that a relationship exists. It is difficult to assess the causality of risk factors in contributing to a problem, as an experimental design is needed – i.e. a controlled study involving randomisation – which has ethical implications when thinking about randomly assigning risk factors to participants.

Grey literature is another type of evidence that can provide useful information about the causes of a problem. Grey literature is any type of literature that is not published in the academic literature. It is usually published by non-research related organisations to share their results for funders, stakeholders and the general public. For instance, if your topic is related to alcohol, you could search the Alcohol Focus Scotland website for relevant resources. A general internet search is also likely to yield relevant results.

Consideration of the quality of the evidence and its relevance to your local context

The context of what you read may differ markedly from the context you wish to implement an intervention in – as such, some of the risk factors and causes that the authors identify may be more, less or not important in your own setting. However, you could use the information to assess (i) if all these risk factors are present in your community, (ii) which are the most important ones in your community (i.e. which factors contribute most to the problem), and (iii) whether there are other important factors in your community which are not included in the scientific evidence.

For example, a key cause of hospital infections in the United States may be poor handwashing technique, but in a country with insufficient healthcare infrastructure, the main cause could be lack of personal protective and sterilising equipment. It would be inappropriate to try to generalise the causes of hospital infection from one context to another as they are less applicable in the other context. If you were to base your intervention development on causes identified in Step 1 that were inappropriate to your setting, you are unlikely to develop an intervention that works.

Historical and cultural factors

The history of a problem can shed light on how it is distributed in the community and what the underlying causal factors are. Examination of this allows for increased understanding of the problem and can shed light on what solutions may be appropriate moving forward. For example, policies that may influence your problem are often due to historical context at the time the policy was implemented – who was in power in the government and their political views, whether there were any conflicts going on, and so on. To understand a problem's history might mean asking some potentially sensitive and difficult questions about what has happened to a community in the past. This should be done with grace and respect, and requires the involvement of stakeholders either through your team or wider stakeholders within the community. Understanding the historical context allows you to approach the problem with cultural sensitivity and greater understanding. This can lead to a more acceptable, sustainable and community-based intervention. You can again use a workshop format to elicit this information, breaking into small groups to discuss the issue and come up with some key issues, and perhaps a timeline of events.

Activity 4.1

Polio Vaccinations

Dr Divya works for a vaccination non-governmental organisation (NGO) and wants to understand why polio vaccination rates are low in a certain part of India. There are many NGOs who have campaigns in the area and the government is very encouraging, but nearly 6% of India's children do not get the four required vaccine doses to protect against polio. Research literature (e.g. epidemiological data, etc) suggests that there may be many reasons for this, including poverty, cultural beliefs, poor medical record-keeping and lack of legislation and infrastructure supporting vaccination. But during the team workshops, some of the stakeholders reveal some worrisome history. Even as recently as the 1970s, forced sterilisations took place in parts of India, making many Indians very wary of government health initiatives. Also, other vaccination campaigns resulted in deaths as vaccines were contaminated and handled improperly. There are still fears today that any government 'help' or assistance is not as benevolent as it seems. For this reason, people are not allowing their children to be vaccinated for polio, which keeps this highly infectious disease endemic in the country. Based on this information, which of the factors influencing vaccination do you think is most important?

Theoretical evidence

Formalised theories can sometimes be valuable in understanding a problem and its causes. For instance, if the problem is a workplace-related health issue, organisational theories can be used to start thinking about how the context of the workplace may influence the problem. Also, when the problem is health behaviour, models of health-related behaviour, such as social cognition models used in the field of health psychology, can sometimes be useful to identify the determinants of the behaviour. However, there have been debates to suggest that some models of health-related behaviour often fail to consistently explain reliable levels of variability between people's behaviours. There are also criticisms that individual-level health behaviour theories do not account for broader, systemic influences on behaviour. But despite their shortcomings, these models are useful

Knowledge link:
This topic is
also covered in
Chapter 6

to prompt thinking about the problem. Chapter 6 discusses how theories may be used to design intervention components to address the problem.

Understanding the nature of the problem: risk factor or outcome

In order to understand the problem, it is important to determine whether the problem is a risk factor for the disease or the condition you are trying to address, or whether it is the actual disease or condition itself. An example of such a public health problem is that of diabetes. Diabetes has many risk factors which interact with each other and can be influenced by broader systems such as the food system, the transport system and the city planning system. All of the risk factors contribute to a greater or lesser extent to the development of diabetes. If you decide to intervene on physical inactivity from a purely individual level, it will not be enough to reduce diabetes if other risk factors (such as the availability of healthy foods) are equally or more important. Therefore, you need to examine the relative importance of physical activity in the midst of several risk factors for diabetes.

In practice, there may be an overlap between risk factors and disease – for example, some people see obesity as a risk factor for other diseases (such as heart disease and diabetes) whereas others consider it as a disease in its own right.

UNDERSTANDING THE SYSTEMS INVOLVED IN THE PROBLEM

In Chapter 2, we introduced the concept of systems and systems thinking. Whilst developing your thinking on the causes of the problem, you and the team may have already started to think about the systems that are influencing the problem and potentially how they interact. Systems thinking can provide a powerful approach to understand the problem and its causes. It focuses on how things are connected to each other; therefore, when considering a problem, systems thinking can help us to consider: (1) the connections between the problem and the systems that affect the problem, (2) the interactions and directionality between the system and the causes of the problem and, ultimately, (3) where an intervention might be made for the greatest impact. For example, the problem of obesity can be conceptualised as an interaction of the food, employment, transport, economic, health and other systems that influence energy intake and expenditure of individuals. Therefore, adopting systems thinking to understand the problem of obesity and its causes will involve carefully reviewing and clarifying the various causes of obesity in each system and understanding how they contribute to the condition of obesity.

Knowledge link: This topic is also covered in Chapter 2

TOOLS FOR DISPLAYING CAUSES OF THE PROBLEM AND RELATED SYSTEMS

Once you and the team have figured out the causes of a problem, it is useful to use diagrams to understand how the various causal factors affect the problem and where along the causal pathways you may be able to intervene.

Mind-maps

The idea behind conducting **mind-mapping** is that each stakeholder or team member will bring their ideas on the topic and discuss them together as a group. As discussed, each stakeholder's perspective around the causes of a problem might be different. Mapping out everyone's views in one place (a whiteboard or large sheet of paper can be helpful) can produce a broader understanding of the causes of the problem. It is important to remember that some causes can be listed in several places if they relate to several key categories. This can generate deeper levels of understanding into the causes of the problem.

One way to undertake a mind-mapping exercise is to hold a workshop in which participants are split into groups, with one group in charge of brainstorming all causal factors related to one category (either a type of system or level of society by theory – for example, the socioecological model). Each group is then asked to mind-map all the possible causes of the problem based on their assigned category, which are then added to an overarching mind-map of all the groups' categories. The whole group then reconvenes to look at the entire mind-map and discusses overlaps, similarities, differences and relationships between the different factors identified.

Diagrams based on the socio-ecological model

The socio-ecological model of health, originally developed by Bronfenbrenner, can be used to categorise causal factors to a problem. The socio-ecological model provides a framework to understand the interplay of key factors at individual, relationship, community and societal levels that influence health, as seen in Figure 4.4 (Whitehead and Dahlgren, 1991).

The factors that influence health can be considered as the causes of the problem, therefore can be mapped onto the socio-ecological model. Figure 4.5 shows an example of how this has been used to understand the causal pathways that affect gender-based violence (Wight et al., 2016).

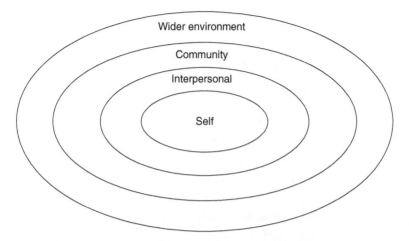

Figure 4.4 The socio-ecological model of health, as developed by Bronfenbrenner

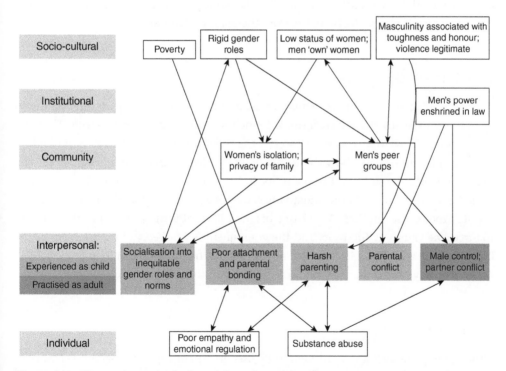

Figure 4.5 The socio-ecological models and causal pathways perpetuating gender-based violence

Source: Wight et al. (2016) (CC BY 4.0)

Fishbone diagrams (cause-and-effect diagrams)

Another visual way of depicting the many possible causes of the problem is by the use of a fishbone/Ishikawa diagram. A **fishbone diagram** is a cause-and-effect diagram used to identify the possible causes of a problem, and facilitates mind-mapping with stakeholders to identify the major categories of causes of a problem. Limitations of fishbone diagrams are that they don't depict causal loops and do not provide explanation of systems that affect the problem.

Figure 4.6 demonstrates how we created a fishbone diagram with stakeholders as part of a project that aimed to develop an intervention to reduce admission to hospitals following intensive care unit (ICU) admission. The development of the fishbone diagram was undertaken as a workshop with stakeholders from all over the UK who have an interest in the problem. Stakeholders were asked to agree on the problem statement. Following a series of group activities, stakeholders agreed the problem statement as 'high readmission rates to hospital in patients with complex health and social needs following intensive care unit admission'. This was captured at the centre of a whiteboard, and a box was drawn around it. A horizontal line from this was then drawn. Inspired by the key categories of the socio-ecological model, stakeholders were grouped into five groups. These key categories are the branches from the main horizontal line.

Root-tree diagrams

A root-tree diagram or root cause analysis is another useful way of analysing the causes of a problem visually. Trees have a trunk, branches, leaves and sometimes fruit. These are the parts of the tree that you see. However, the roots are buried in the soil or ground. In order to truly understand how the trunk, branches, leaves and fruit are supported, you need to dig into the soil to get to the roots. In the same way, you need to dig deep down on an issue to fully unearth the underlying causes of a problem. That is why this approach is called root cause analysis. A root-tree diagram illustrates the problem as the trunk of the tree, the causes as the roots and the consequences or effects of the problem as the branches or leaves. This pictorial way of teasing out the problem can help you establish causal pathways and enhance your understanding of the causes of the problem.

Logic models

Knowledge link: This topic is also covered in Chapter 6, 7 and 10

Although logic models are more commonly used in visualising the programme theory of an intervention, they can also be used to depict cause and effect. Figure 4.7 demonstrates how a logic model has been used to demonstrate the causal pathways to poor HIV treatment and prevention outcomes. This example is part of the case study carried out by Masquillier et al. (2020), presented in Chapter 10.

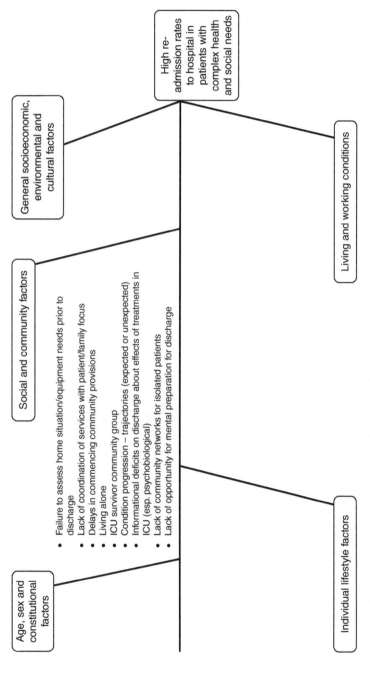

Figure 4.6 Using a fishbone diagram to develop an intervention to reduce admission to hospital following intensive care unit (ICU) admission

Age, sex and constitutional factors

Social and community factors

General socioeconomic, environmental and cultural factors

High re-admission rates to hospital in patients with complex health and social needs

- Failure to assess home situation/equipment needs prior to discharge
- Lack of coordination of services with patient/family focus
- Delays in commencing community provisions
- Living alone
- ICU survivor community group
- Condition progression – trajectories (expected or unexpected)
- Informational deficits on discharge about effects of treatments in ICU (esp. psychobiological)
- Lack of community networks for isolated patients
- Lack of opportunity for mental preparation for discharge

Living and working conditions

Individual lifestyle factors

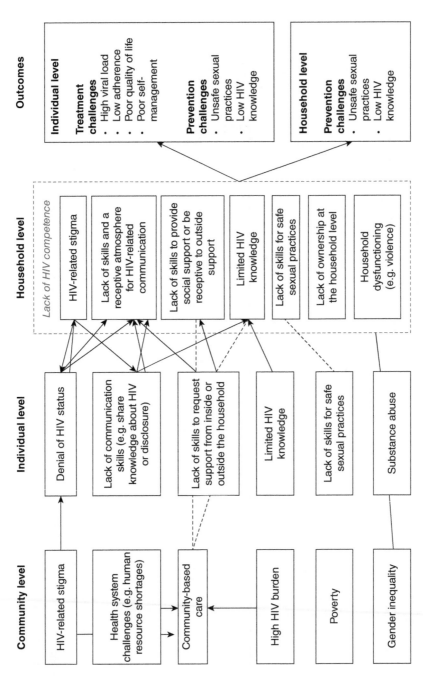

Figure 4.7 A logic model demonstrating causal pathways to poor HIV treatment and prevention outcomes

Source: Masquillier et al, (2020) (CC BY)

Causal loop diagrams

Causal loop diagrams can be used to show the relationships between causal factors and how they operate within a system (or systems); Chapter 3 provides one example of a causal loop diagram in relation to COVID-19. There are several ways of developing such diagrams using the methods described above. Another useful worked example, using a systems dynamic approach and focusing on obesity in youth, was undertaken by Waterlander et al. (2020). They developed a causal loop diagram which consisted of multiple subsystems and three types of dynamics appeared, including (1) feedback loops, (2) connections between feedback loops and subsystems, and (3) mechanisms. The process enabled them to identify a range of systems impacting on obesity from the well-known ones such as home and school environments to those less often focused on such as macroeconomics, social welfare and urban systems.

Knowledge link: This topic is also covered in Chapter 3

SUMMARY

This chapter has covered the first step of the 6SQuID framework: understanding the problem and its causes. A number of issues have been discussed, such as ensuring that stakeholders agree on the definition of the problem. Early agreement will make later stages of the intervention development process go more smoothly, as stakeholders will have a common understanding of what exactly the intervention will be addressing.

A workshop format is strongly encouraged as a good way of undertaking activities with your stakeholders to define and understand the problem. Some of the tools you could use to do this are rich pictures, multi-perspective approach diagrams and world cafes. It is also important to have a thorough understanding of the potential causes of the problem, the systems they operate in and their contribution to the problem. There are many different data sources you could use to undertake this exercise, such as epidemiological evidence, which may be captured in a systematic review, and formalised theories such as models of health-related behaviours, if the problem is behaviour-related. These sources of evidence from academic or grey literature may be generic and may need to be understood within your local context as part of workshop activities with stakeholders.

It is useful in Step 1 to outline how the various causal pathways affect the problem diagrammatically. With this being done, you can then begin to think about how to assess which of the factors could be modified and those that are likely to have the maximum effects if modified through an intervention. The next chapter goes into far more depth with this and will help you decide how important each cause is, and whether or not it can be changed (if it's *modifiable or non-modifiable*), but considering this early when generating a list or diagram of causes for a problem is helpful.

FURTHER READING

Funnell, S. C., and Rogers, P. J. (2011) *Purposeful Program Theory: Effective Use of Theories of Change and Logic Models*, vol. 31. Chichester: John Wiley & Sons.

Waterlander, W. E., Singh, A., Altenburg, T., et al. (2020) 'Understanding obesity-related behaviors in youth from a systems dynamics perspective: the use of causal loop diagrams', *Obesity Reviews, 22* (7): e13185. https://doi.org/10.1111/obr.13185

REFERENCES

Bradshaw, J. (1972) 'A taxonomy of social need', in G. McLachlan (ed.), *Problems and Progress in Medical Care*. 7th series. Buckingham: NPHT/Open University Press.

Checkland, P. (2000) 'Soft systems methodology: a thirty year retrospective', *Systems Research, 17*: S11–S58. https://doi.org/10.1002/1099-1743(200011)17:1+<::AID-SRES374>3.0.CO;2-O

Green, L. W., and Kreuter, M. W. (2005) *Precede-Proceed. Health Program Planning: An Educational and Ecological Approach*, 4th edn. New York: McGraw-Hill.

Masquillier, C., Wouters, E., Campbell, L., Delport, A., Sematlane, N., Dube, L., and Knight, L. (2020) Households in HIV care: designing an intervention to stimulate HIV competency in households in South Africa. *Frontiers in Public Health, 8*: 246. doi: 10.3389/fpubh.2020.00246

Morgan, P. I., and Ogbonna, E. (2008) 'Subcultural dynamics in transformation: A multi-perspective study of healthcare professionals', *Human Relations, 61* (1): 39–65. doi:10.1177/0018726707085945

Waterlander, W. E., Singh, A., Altenburg, T., et al. (2020) 'Understanding obesity-related behaviors in youth from a systems dynamics perspective: the use of causal loop diagrams', *Obesity Reviews, 22* (7): e13185. https://doi.org/10.1111/obr.13185

Whitehead, M., and Dahlgren, G. (1991) 'What can be done about inequalities in health?', *The Lancet, 338*: 1059–63. doi:10.1016/0140-6736(91)91911-D

Wight, D., Wimbush, E., Jepson, R., and Doi, L. (2016) 'Six steps in quality intervention development (6SQuID)', *Journal of Epidemiology and Community Health, 70*: 520–5.

ACTIVITY ANSWERS

Scenario 4.1: A community gambling problem

Jendyose

1. What exactly is the problem? Is it the gambling itself, or the consequences of the gambling? After all, not all people who gamble run into difficulties.

2. What are the main causes of the problem? Which groups are most affected by the problem?
3. Which are the main systems that influence the problem? Is it just the gambling industry or are there other systems involved?
4. How did did the problem start?
5. Why does the problem exist?

Activity 4.1: Polio vaccinations

Dr Divya and her team decide that historical lack of trust in the government is a key factor in low vaccination rates. This may be a more important factor than any that were found in the epidemiological evidence. They begin to explore more about the history of the lack of trust: how it came about, why it has continued into recent times and so on before considering if this is a modifiable problem, as the next chapter will cover.

5
6SQUID STEP 2: IDENTIFYING MODIFIABLE CAUSAL FACTORS

Learning objectives

After reading this chapter, you will be able to:

- Understand the differences between modifiable, hard to modify and non-modifiable factors
- Clarify which causal or contextual factors are modifiable and have greatest scope for change
- Understand how to select which factor/s to target.

Scenario 5.1

Sleep problems

Bella has been struggling to sleep during the hot summer months. As a result, she is making numerous errors in her day job as a financial auditor for a large company and is finding it increasingly difficult to concentrate. She is feeling exhausted as a result. She realises that she must address the issue before it damages her health and affects her work performance.

To find a solution, she creates a list of all the possible causes for her sleep issues. Looking at her list, she decides that there are certain factors that are within her direct control to change (**modifiable factors**), some that she may have limited control over changing (**hard to modify factors**) and some that are outside of her control (**non-modifiable factors**). Bella thinks about which factors she could change in order to resolve her sleep issues. She groups them into the categories shown in Table 5.1.

Table 5.1   Modifiable, hard to modify and non-modifiable factors associated with sleep problems

Modifiable	Hard to modify	Non-modifiable
Checking work emails at night in bed	Workplace stress	8-month-old daughter teething and crying
Too much screen time before and whilst in bed	Noise from next-door neighbours	Partner away overseas working
Working on her laptop in bed at night	Feeling too hot (recent heatwave)	
Coffee and/or wine before bed		

How might Bella change those factors listed as modifiable and hard to modify? What challenges might she encounter? For each of the two non-modifiable factors, explain why these cannot be changed.

INTRODUCTION

Reflection on the causes of a problem is necessary to maximise the chances of an intervention succeeding. For example, one of our co-authors has an unused gym membership. To increase usage of the gym membership, our colleague needs to consider what is causing the problem, and think about how to intervene. Are there any factors they could easily modify such as their motivation? Are any harder to modify, such as transport to the gym which is some miles away? What is non-modifiable and outside of their control, such as the limited opening times of the gym? One of the key mistakes in intervention development is that people move too quickly towards the intervention stage without fully considering the modifiable, hard to modify and non-modifiable factors contributing to the problem. This may result in interventions which are ineffective because they targeted the wrong causal factor(s), so a change in the outcome could never hope to be achieved. By now you may have identified the causal factors and have visualised these using one of the methods described in Chapter 4. To move forward, it is necessary to decide which factor or factors you intend to target as part of your intervention. This is the first step towards identifying how to create change and represents a critical moment in

Knowledge link:
This topic is
also covered in
Chapter 4

the intervention development process. Decisions at this stage will provide the foundation upon which your intervention will be developed and will ensure that you are in a good position moving forward.

Knowledge link: This topic is also covered in Chapter 4

Many factors combine to affect the health of individuals and communities: politics, policy and legislation; where we live, work and play; environmental and geographical conditions; individual characteristics such as behaviour, beliefs and genetic makeup, income and education level; and relationships with one another. These factors also interact with one another and exist within systems. Some of these are outside of the direct control of anyone. It is important to identify and consider all factors that may contribute to the problem you have chosen to target and to think about which are within your scope to intervene upon. But a word of caution. Just because they are within your control to intervene on, does not mean that they are the most important or will solve the problem. For example, our co-author may become very motivated to use the gym by using a goal-setting intervention, but still cannot get to the gym because they don't have transport.

Knowledge link: This topic is also covered in Chapter 3

Activity 5.1

Reflection

Think about a problem you have currently, e.g. lack of sleep, lack of exercise. Write down all the potential factors that may be contributing to the problem. If you wish, use a diagram to illustrate the relationships between them. Identify which factors you think might be easy, hard or impossible to change. Once you have done this, try to identify the factors you think need to be addressed to have the biggest impact upon the problem. Are they mainly easy, hard or impossible to change?

Knowledge link: This topic is also covered in Chapter 4

MODIFIABLE, HARD TO MODIFY AND NON-MODIFIABLE FACTORS

A **modifiable factor** is a risk factor that can be changed and controlled to some extent. This is easily illustrated using a biomedical example, as shown in Figure 5.1. Cardiovascular disease (CVD) is influenced by many factors that can be controlled through medication and behavioural changes, for example high blood pressure and lack of physical activity. These factors are considered modifiable as they are amenable to change, i.e. these factors could be changed by providing high blood pressure medication alongside support for making behavioural changes to result in increased physical activity. However, a number of factors remain that are **non-modifiable**, such as many genetic factors and age. These would be almost impossible to change – as much as some of us might like to change our age, this factor will remain non-modifiable until the fountain of youth is discovered.

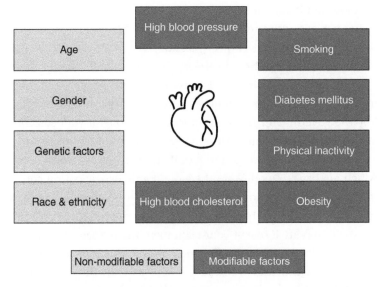

Figure 5.1   Modifiable and non-modifiable factors in cardiovascular disease

You may have noticed that the factors in Figure 5.1 are all at the level of the individual (more proximal). However, it is rarely this simple in public health. Contributing factors in public health exist at many different levels (both proximal and distal). Take the example of tobacco use in young people. This problem is not a medical condition, but a behaviour embedded within specific social and environmental contexts and systems. Figure 5.2 illustrates some of the causal factors relating to this problem.

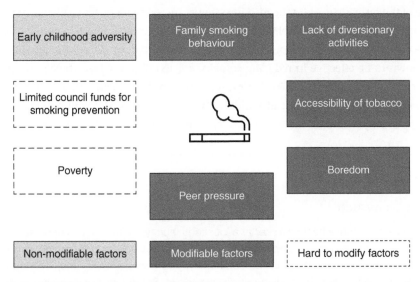

Figure 5.2   Modifiable and non-modifiable factors in tobacco use in young people

In this example, modifiable factors exist at the individual level (boredom); family level (family smoking behaviour); community level (lack of diversionary activities and accessibility of tobacco); and social level (peer pressure). A further two factors exist that can be categorised as **hard to modify**. In theory, it is possible to change these, however, in practice, this is likely to be difficult. For example, both poverty and limited council funds for smoking prevention work could be addressed in legislative or budgetary changes introduced by the government. However, unless you or one of your stakeholders are in government and/or in a powerful position (e.g. the UK prime minister with a majority backing), these things will remain hard to modify (but are always worth considering).

Factors which are hard to modify are therefore highly dependent on context, and the extent to which you will be able to target these depends to some extent on the stakeholder makeup of the team developing the intervention. For example, lack of diversionary activities may be easier to modify if one of your team members is a senior member of the local council community planning partnership. Such a person may be able to divert existing resources to create these activities or introduce these activities into an existing local community initiative. You may also consider whether there are local assets such as youth groups and approach them to join your team. The factor may then become easier to modify.

Knowledge link:
This topic is
also covered in
Chapter 3

Non-modifiable factors and their potential effect must always be considered, regardless of whether these are within your reach as an intervention developer. In this example, adverse childhood experiences may increase the risk of a child taking up smoking. There is little you can do about this non-modifable factor, but it is useful to keep this in mind and understand its contribution to the problem.

Knowledge link:
This topic is
also covered in
Chapter 6

Proximal factors are those that are closer to the individual and therefore more immediately amenable to change (e.g. attitudes and beliefs). **Distal factors** are those that exist outside of the individual, are embedded in systems, and present greater challenge in terms of intervention (e.g. poverty). Despite the greater challenge, interventions targeting distal factors are often highly effective. For example, legislation to ban smoking in public places has been shown to be effective in reducing smoking-related illness. Given the complexity and number of causal factors underpinning most public health problems, an effective intervention should attempt to intervene at multiple levels. The next section will provide guidance related to issues you should consider when you are deciding which factors to target.

Activity 5.2

Decision making

Lewis is a community health worker at a local community centre. He has been asked by the lead health worker to establish a project team and to develop a community intervention to improve low mood in the community. The community is rural, isolated and has recently experienced flooding due to heavy rain. Some community members have

reported feeling lonely and at a loss for what to do, due to a lack of activities and facilities in town. Unfortunately, the community centre has been closed for a year due to local
government funding cuts. Due to the time of year, the town is dark from 4pm till 8am the
following day. Lewis will develop the intervention with a group of community representatives and a junior member of the local council.

Draw a diagram showing what you think are the modifiable, hard to modify and non-
modifiable factors.

PRIORITISING WHICH MODIFIABLE FACTORS TO TARGET

The next stage for your team is to choose which factors to target; a process that involves
prioritising those factors you have identified. This decision will guide the remainder of
the intervention development process. The factors you select will provide the building
blocks of your intervention going forward. It is therefore critical that you consider all relevant information at this stage. For this section, we will use the example problem of school
absenteeism, which places children at risk of developing unhealthy behaviours in adolescence and young adulthood as well as having implications for their health in later life.
Figure 5.3 illustrates some of the modifiable, hard to modify and non-modifiable factors
relating to this problem. These include modifiable factors at the school level (poor teaching, lack of school-based initiatives); family level (poor parental monitoring); individual

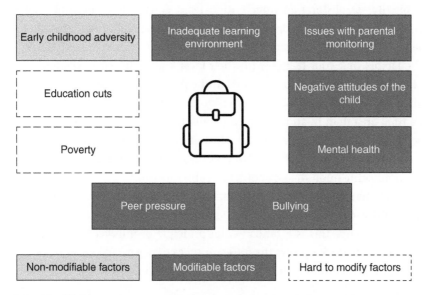

Figure 5.3   Modifiable and non-modifiable factors in school absenteeism

level (negative attitudes towards school, substance misuse); and peer level (bullying). We will also introduce a useful priority exercise intervention development tool.

The decision on which factors to prioritise should be guided by consideration of the following: (1) which factors contribute most to the problem in your local context, (2) the available resources, (3) the systems in which you wish to implement your intervention, and (4) ethics and acceptability.

Identifying the contribution of factors in your local context

The extent to which each factor contributes to the problem has to be considered. It is unlikely that all factors are equally important, with some playing a more important role than others. To identify the relative importance of each factor, you should draw upon the local knowledge and contextual experience of your team and wider stakeholders, and any existing evidence.

Using local knowledge and contextual experience to inform the contribution of factors

Throughout this book, we emphasise the importance of local knowledge and contextual experience. This is the bedrock of intervention development since such knowledge and experience increase the likelihood of your intervention being acceptable, effective and sustainable. By establishing an intervention team consisting of multiple stakeholders, you will have access to knowledge and experience that can guide decisions around which modifiable factors could and should be targeted to effect change in that specific con-

Knowledge link: This topic is also covered in Chapter 2

text. The factors that your team – with their local knowledge and experience – uncover may differ from any factors you identified in the published literature or your pre-existing assumptions. For example, transport provision may contribute more to school absenteeism in a rural area than in an urban area. Similarly, having to provide financially for an extended family may be of little relevance in some countries but a major factor in others. Table 5.2 shows an example of how context may influence the relative contribution of parental monitoring upon the issue of school absenteeism.

We propose that you draw upon the local knowledge and contextual experience of both your team and wider stakeholders. The identification of which factors to target should be co-produced, since this is a fundamental principle of intervention development. To illustrate this, Scenario 5.2 shows the different types of perspectives that stakeholders can bring to the decision around which modifiable factors to target in the example of school absenteeism.

Knowledge link: This topic is also covered in Chapter 2

Table 5.2   Example of how context may influence the relative contribution of parental monitoring on the issue of school absenteeism

Context	Example	Effect on the relative contribution of the factor
Demographics	Number of single parents	May be more of a factor in large families
	Number of children in family	
Geography	Distance from school	Parent may find it harder to monitor children who go to school a long way away
Culture	Expectations of parenting	Different cultures may have different approaches
Politics	Budget allocation to schools and communities	Different areas may receive different levels of funding for parent support services

Scenario 5.2

Stakeholder perspectives on school absenteeism

Jan was asked to develop a school absenteeism intervention for young people in the local community. She has received some funding from the local authority. Jan reached out to stakeholders who now comprise her project team. Her team includes secondary school pupils, teachers, a member of the education authority and a parent group.

Ahmed, Marc and Megan – secondary school pupils

Ahmed, Marc and Megan are sixth-form pupils who have set up a peer mentoring service within the local secondary school. The service is aimed at any pupil who is struggling with coursework, or with any other problem that may directly affect their wellbeing. During the establishment of this service, they spoke with pupils about the type of issues affecting them. These included in-school and online bullying, issues with teachers and lack of engaging material during class. Additionally, issues around substance abuse were reported. Ahmed, Marc and Megan can advise on factors as they specifically relate to the context of the school environment. As pupils, they also have knowledge of the school system.

Susan – member of the education authority

Susan is the education officer for the area. Her role involves monitoring school performance, including quality of teaching and number of school absences. Susan is a member of the oversight group for developing the national curriculum, and as such is well connected to government leads in this area. Whilst she does not work directly with young people, she is well placed to make a judgement as to the local political, funding and practical issues. Susan has knowledge of the education system at both at a local and a national level.

(Continued)

George, Mei Xing, Claire and John – teachers

The teachers have a keen interest in the issue of school absenteeism and have formed a school committee to tackle this. They are collecting data on the prevalence of absenteeism in the school and have conducted a small research project with teachers as to what is causing the issue. They have also noted an increase in reports of online and in-school bullying. The teaching staff can advise on the factors from a teachers' perspective. They have knowledge of the school system.

Ali and Priya – parents

Ali and Priya were nominated by a parents' group to represent them on the team. Through conversations over the past few years, pressing issues regarding the learning experience have been brought to the fore. They feel that these issues are most certainly contributing to the problem of school absenteeism. Ali and Priya can advise on the factors from a parents' perspective. They have some knowledge of the school system.

In Scenario 5.2, Jan has set up a team that has local knowledge and contextual experience in relation to school absenteeism. Working with her team, she can conduct a prioritisation exercise to identify which modifiable factors they should target as part of their intervention.

INTERVENTION DEVELOPMENT TOOL: CONTEXT MAPPING

A useful tool for understanding more about the opportunities or constraints of your local context is through context mapping (Jan could do this with her group). It can help you understand more about which factors can be controlled or influenced; what constrains your options and/or actions; and what potential assets there are. It challenges assumptions around what you really have the power to influence and can help you identify other stakeholders you may need to engage with to make change happen.

You can do this activity either face to face or online with your stakeholder group. In preparation, draw three concentric ellipses of increasing size, as shown in Figure 5.4, and label them as in the figure. More detail is provided below:

1. Central ellipse: the factor (or stakeholder, organisation, system) is within the remit or control of one or more stakeholders in the group.
2. The factor (or stakeholder, organisation, system) is part of/relevant to your situation, but is not under your control/authority; you might be able to or may need to influence it.

3. The factor is a constraint on what you can do or how you can act. You may recognise that you need to be able to influence it and, therefore, identify it as something to be moved into one of the inner circles.
4. Fuzzy outer region: national or global constraints – often legislation/regulation/political/environmental.

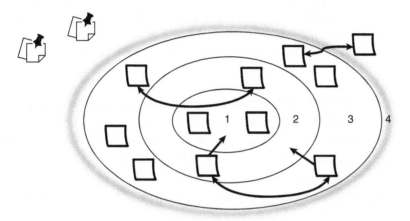

1. Factors within the control of your team
2. Factors you can/may need to influence
3. Situational constraints
4. Standing constraints

Figure 5.4   Context mapping

Make sure that participants have access either to sticky notes or some way of writing on an online board. Then ask the stakeholders to write down all your factors and place them in one of the rings. For those factors placed in rings 2 or 3, what would be needed to move them into the central ellipse? Is there someone you can ask to join the stakeholder group, for example? What influence is needed, and is it something that is possible within the team? You can refer back to any of the diagrams you have created earlier to help with this exercise.

INTERVENTION DEVELOPMENT TOOL: PRIORITISATION EXERCISE

A prioritisation exercise essentially involves working with a group (in-person or online) to reach a consensus. This exercise is best done as a group rather than individually since a group-based format encourages discussion and exchange of ideas between individuals bringing different local and contextual experience. Essentially this involves:

- Generating a list of factors from those involved via small group discussion and brainstorming
- Discussion of the relevance of any factors you uncover in the existing evidence of your local context (next section)
- Discussion and agreement on which factors are modifiable and which are within the reasonable scope of those involved in the team to change.
- Prioritisation of modifiable factors by asking the group to vote using stickies or some other such method and asking them to place these beside those factors that they consider to be most important.
- Discussion of the final list of prioritised factors and refinements agreed by consensus if necessary.

Additional information may be brought to the fore during this exercise that requires you to revisit any context mapping you have conducted and to rethink the composition of your team. For example, you may identify a modifiable factor operating in a system for which you do not have any current representation on your team. You may decide as a group that it would be worthwhile to reach out to someone who could represent this system, thereby potentially opening an avenue to targeting this factor as part of your intervention.

Activity 5.3

Planning

Plan a workshop for Jan in Scenario 5.2, outlining a prioritisation exercise to identify which modifiable factors to target. Specify:

- Who you would invite to the workshop and why
- The factors you think they might consider to be most important based on information provided in the scenario
- Activities you would use to reach consensus (feel free to use activities presented elsewhere in the book, since they can be used across chapters).

USING EVIDENCE TO INFORM THE CONTRIBUTION OF FACTORS

It is useful to identify whether there is any existing available evidence to highlight the contribution of modifiable factors to the problem. This may involve looking at published academic research in addition to local data. Findings can be brought to the group prioritisation exercise outlined previously for discussion around its relevance to the local context.

Published academic research can provide a general indication of the contribution of each factor to the problem. A useful starting point is to identify any relevant literature reviews that have attempted to synthesise observational studies. These studies gather data related to a specific problem and attempt to quantify the extent to which they influence or predict that problem. It is likely that someone else will have looked broadly and comprehensively across this literature, saving you a lot of work in the process. For those of you in academia, literature search tools and electronic access to journals are readily available. For those of you outside academia, a Google search will often suffice for a broad overview. Many papers are open access (i.e. freely available), with authors often posting pre-print copies of their work on research websites such as ResearchGate (www.researchgate.net). Alternatively, you may find useful summaries of the literature to guide your decision making on the websites of most major health bodies, for example the National Health Service, the National Institute for Health and the World Health Organisation.

In relation to the problem in Scenario 5.2, a search of the published literature relating to school absenteeism identifies a review by Gubbels et al. (2019). The authors report a **meta-analysis**, which is a statistical method of combining data from multiple studies. Seventy-five studies were included in that report on 781 potential risk factors for school absenteeism. Compared to the six factors listed in Figure 5.3, the comparably high number of 781 factors identified by the reviewers gives you some indication of exactly how complex these types of issues can be. The authors identified factors that had medium to large effects on the problem, including two of those shown in Figure 5.3 – substance misuse and negative attitudes towards school. This is helpful to know, but as we have outlined, it should not be the sole source of information from which you select your modifiable targets. This is because this literature reports work undertaken in many different contexts. In this case, the 75 included studies were conducted in different countries, schools and environmental settings. It is worth noting that what is important in one context may not be as important in another. Therefore, whilst it is certainly valuable to note that the research evidence supports the idea that absenteeism is encouraged by negative attitudes towards school and substance misuse, it is necessary to consider the extent to which this applies to your local context.

Local data refer to any data that is specific to the local context in which your intervention is to be implemented. This could be routine data such as service evaluations or performance and monitoring reports, or data specific to the local community provided by national health bodies. For example, in Scotland, the Scottish Government and the National Health Service (NHS) publish figures related to various health-related outcomes, broken down by local authority. In Scenario 5.2, the teachers who are participating in the team have collected data on the prevalence of absenteeism and have conducted a small qualitative project with colleagues as to what they think is causing the issue. These are local data.

To some extent, the presence of local data enables examination of the problem in a specific context. However, it is important to note that such data are not always available and sometimes data that are particularly useful may not be reported. The key is to look at both forms of evidence, if possible, drawing upon research and local data alongside a prioritisation exercise to draw upon local knowledge and contextual experience.

THEORY OF CAUSES: HOW CAUSAL FACTORS RELATE TO ONE ANOTHER

Knowledge link: This topic is also covered in Chapter 3

Causal factors exist within a system. It is not possible to understand the problem or its parts in isolation. In a system, all factors are related. It is the relationships between factors that cause the problem and therefore it is important to consider how factors relate to one another when selecting which to target. It is likely that targeting some modifiable factors may result in an indirect knock-on effect upon others. These can be referred to as clusters of factors. The relationship between causal factors as they exist within system/s and their role in influencing the problem, can be described as a **theory of causes** (Komro, 2018). In an ideal situation, you would aim to impact upon as many of these factors as possible to give your intervention the best chance of success. Figure 5.5 illustrates this in relation to school absenteeism.

In this example, targeting two modifiable factors will likely result in indirect results upon three additional modifiable factors. Targeting the learning environment may result in positive attitudes towards school. Similarly, targeting bullying may result in more positive attitudes, better mental health and less substance use, all of which have an effect on absenteeism. This example shows that it is important to think about how factors cluster and relate to one another.

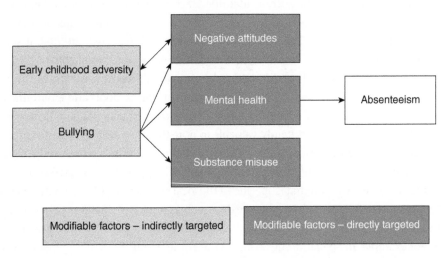

Figure 5.5   Simplified theory of causes showing modifiable factors in school absenteeism

THE FACTORS YOU TARGET SHOULD BE GUIDED BY YOUR AVAILABLE RESOURCES

The available resources will have a major influence upon your decision making in terms of which factors to target. A resource is any tangible or non-tangible support that could be called upon or used in the intervention development process. These can be categorised in terms of who is involved in your project and what skills or access they can offer, and what physical resources are available to you (such as funding, staff time, venues). Another way to conceptualise resources is to think of them as assets that will increase the likelihood of success in tackling the problem. These can be:

Knowledge link: This topic is also covered in Chapter 2

- Economic, e.g. funding
- Physical, e.g. environmental, space
- Community, e.g. local groups, existing infrastructure, community members
- Human resources within a system, e.g. capacity, time, staff
- Cultural, e.g. faith-based organisations, cultural values
- Stakeholders.

Economic resources

In Scenario 5.2, Jan's team received funding for the project. The trouble is that most funding is short-term and they only received a limited amount. If the team is relying solely on that funding, then the project will be short-term. By co-producing her intervention, her team – which consists of individuals from quite different backgrounds – may be able to provide funding solutions that she herself may not have been able to access.

Physical resources

Jan's team must consider what physical resources are available – for example, if there is space within the school or the local community that could be utilised. By co-producing the intervention with the input of teachers and someone from the education authority, Jan could work to embed any intervention within existing systems, for instance school routines.

Community resources

The team could investigate if there are any local groups to support their anti-bullying initiatives that could be a resource for them as the project moves forward. They could invite a representative from such a group to be part of the project team, thereby potentially drawing upon additional existing resources (as well as further valuable knowledge and experience). They should also consider the wider knowledge, skills and lived experience available within the community and draw upon this.

Human resources

Many interventions require some form of human resource to deliver. It may be that teachers are already overcommitted and may not be able to fit another activity into their daily routine. However, there may be some capacity within a group of teachers for whom this topic is a professional interest. By co-producing the intervention, individuals who make up the team may also be able to offer solutions to this – for example, perhaps they are able to spare a member of staff for a number of hours per week.

Cultural

The team might be able to identify some faith-based and cultural groups who are interested in the topic area and able to provide resources from time to funding.

Stakeholders

Jan has access to teachers and a member of the Education Authority, which immediately opens doors for her in terms of considering intervening upon school factors such as poor teaching and lack of school-based initiatives. If she did not have these contacts, intervening at the school level would be difficult. How would she gain access to schools? How could she identify what is missing currently in terms of school-based initiatives? How would she ensure her ideas are implemented?

The available resources will influence the decision as to which factors to select. If you are lucky enough to have some funding, it is prudent to think sensibly about how to get the most out of this. People often spend money on the things that are least likely to have an impact (e.g. leaflet campaigns). It is important to spend such funding on activities that are likely to be effective.

SOME FACTORS MAY INTRODUCE ETHICAL CONCERNS

Knowledge link: This topic is also covered in Chapters 2, 6 and 7

Ethical concerns can arise at the point of selecting factors to target for intervention. As stated previously, ethics refers to a system of moral principles which we use to guide our decision making as we navigate the process of intervention development, and is one of our underlying principles of intervention development.

The issue of the measles, mumps and rubella (MMR) vaccination illustrates some of the ethical issues that can occur when deciding which factors to target (in this case, to increase uptake of the vaccine). MMR is the combined vaccination that protects against measles, mumps and rubella. Vaccination offers the safest means of protection. A key factor influencing uptake is parental decision making, itself influenced by additional factors including individual attitudes, knowledge and beliefs, alongside environmental factors such as opportunity and access. Due to a now discredited study published in the late 1990s, concerns regarding the safety of the vaccine – specifically claims linking it to autism – entered the public discourse, influencing many parents' decision as to whether to vaccinate their child. This is despite clear evidence that MMR does not cause autism. As a public health planner at the highest levels of government, it would be possible to remove parental decision making entirely as an influencing factor and introduce legislation to make MMR vaccination compulsory for all children. Whilst this would likely result in more children being vaccinated, questions could be raised as to whether this might encroach upon human rights, i.e. the right of a parent to choose what is best for their child. How do you think parents would feel if this occurred? This might have unintentional consequences, such as increased distrust in government or conspiratorial thinking (Gardner et al., 2010). There is a need for balance between what we know might be a solution to a problem and how that solution might affect those who receive the intervention.

Interventions at all levels, from the individual to the environmental and socioeconomic levels, have ethical implications. However, it could be argued that the more distal the factor you are targeting, the greater the likelihood of such implications. Let's take the example of unhealthy eating habits to illustrate this. One of the factors influencing this is individual choice. This factor could be targeted at the individual level by the application of behaviour change techniques such as dietary planning. Engagement with such techniques requires voluntary participation by an individual, i.e. they must choose to engage with the intervention. Now imagine at the community level, the local council decides to ask large local supermarkets to rearrange food so that healthy options are more visible. There is less individual choice here to take part in the intervention. Finally, imagine that the government bans certain foods from supermarkets. In this example, the whole population take part in the intervention, whether they like it or not, and choice is completely removed as a factor.

Ethical decisions are not clear cut, as quite often the benefits outweigh the costs involved in such interventions. Many of the most successful recent public health interventions have targeted distal factors, through legislation or large-scale change in socioeconomic factors. Such an approach is generally accepted to have the greatest potential for improving health (Frieden, 2010). For example, in 2006, the Scottish Government introduced a smoking ban in public places. This resulted in reduced rates of smoking, fewer young people taking up the habit, changed attitudes towards smoking and bar workers becoming healthier. However, the ban was not welcomed by all, with smokers' rights groups campaigning that it impinged upon smokers' right to choose. In 2020, legislative interventions aimed at reducing the spread of coronavirus were adopted worldwide, including legislation restricting social gatherings, the amount of time people could spend outside their homes and closure of facilities. These interventions were hugely successful; however, similar ethical concerns were raised by some groups. It is therefore important to consider each intervention on a case-by-case basis.

Some 'politically unpalatable' solutions have been implemented successfully, but tend to be instigated by more socially liberal governments. For example, in Scotland the national government introduced a minimum unit pricing for alcohol. However, these examples are few and far between and the term 'nanny state' is often used in such circumstances.

SOME SOLUTIONS MAY BE POLITICALLY UNPALATABLE

Much of what we do in public health exists, or is influenced by, political systems and ideology. The process of selecting which factors to target, therefore, may need to take into account who is in power. Depending on the politics of both national and local government, it may be difficult to address some factors. This is because the act of intervening upon those factors can be seen to be politically undesirable. For example, poverty is one of the main determinants of ill health. Most governments realise this, but few governments would directly improve the financial position of people to impact outcomes such as smoking and obesity. Improving the financial position of members of the population could have a huge positive impact upon health. However, political considerations such as the impact on the wider economy, and public opinion may discount this factor as an option for intervention.

The preference of governments, historically, has been to focus resources upon individual-level interventions. Such interventions place responsibility on individuals and minimise government involvement. However, they are also less effective and may have no to little impact on health inequalities. The approach outlined in this book is that targeting factors at multiple levels will increase the likelihood of intervention success and reduce the likelihood that an intervention will widen health inequalities.

ISSUES TO LOOK OUT FOR AT THIS STAGE

A number of issues exist in relation to this stage of the intervention development process, including the temptation to go for an easy solution, and focusing on single proximal factors. These stem from a fundamental misunderstanding of the nature of public health problems. Developing effective interventions for complex problems in our complex world is not an easy task. There is often a tendency to try to identify a simple solution or a 'quick fix' – quickly intervening around a proximal cause, without stopping to think about the distal systemic cause. Unfortunately, this is not how public health problems work. Complex problems require careful thought and consideration. As explained, such problems exist within a system (or systems); therefore, attempts to intervene should draw upon a full understanding of how causal factors relate to one another within that system.

Knowledge link: This topic is also covered in Chapter 3

Focusing solely on targeting factors at one level

Focusing only upon one level of intervention does not account for the multifaceted nature of public health problems. In order to give your intervention the best chance of success, it is necessary to target factors at multiple levels in multiple different systems. Let's revisit the problem of school absenteeism to illustrate this (see Figure 5.5).

If Jan's team chooses to focus solely on the individual level by targeting negative attitudes towards school and chooses to ignore the school-level factors, it is unlikely that the intervention will have much success. By failing to tackle factors occurring within the school system itself (the poor learning experience and bullying), they have failed to maximise the impact of the intervention by ignoring relationships between these factors and negative attitudes. Similarly, if they choose to focus solely at the school level by improving the learning experience for pupils, they will be ignoring the role of bullying in affecting negative attitudes, mental health and substance use. Note that this relationship is bi-directional, meaning that the two levels influence one another. For their intervention to have the best chance of success, they should target factors at both individual and school levels.

Focusing on increasing awareness and education only

Following on from this, it can be tempting to decide to focus upon the individual level only by increasing education and awareness. The assumption of such interventions is that the main casual factor for almost any problem is lack of awareness and knowledge. However, there is a large body of research demonstrating that the provision of education and raising of awareness – e.g. through leaflets, posters – in isolation of other strategies, are ineffective. This is hardly surprising given that knowledge and awareness are rarely the only factors involved in complex problems such as obesity, partner violence or school absenteeism.

Hillsdon et al. (2002) conducted a randomised controlled trial of 1,658 middle-aged men and women to examine the effectiveness of brief advice from a GP to take more exercise upon physical activity. The intervention participants were given advice about the importance of physical activity as part of their daily routine. In other words, they were provided with education only. There was no difference between the intervention and control groups in level of self-reported physical activity at 12 months. Why might this be the case? We know that physical activity is a complex behaviour influenced by multiple different factors. Causal factors exist at the individual (attitudes, behaviour, etc.), social (peer behaviour, social support, etc.) and community (facilities, opportunity and access, etc.) levels, and in the wider policy context (physical activity legislation dictating funding and priorities for local councils). The suggestion that simply providing someone with information would be enough to create change ignores the complexity at play here. In this example, patients may have absorbed the advice provided to them, but after leaving the surgery become subject to forces outside of their control. Perhaps they cannot get childcare, making it difficult for them to get out and exercise. Perhaps they do not have the funds to travel to the local park or to use swimming facilities. Perhaps there is high crime in the area and there is a fear of exercising outdoors. Perhaps they do not like exercising alone and have few friends. Perhaps the local council has closed crucial local facilities that would have made exercise more accessible for them had they remained open. The list could go on.

Focusing on behaviours without paying attention to the context and systems in which they occur

Knowledge link: This topic is also covered in Chapters 2 and 3

Developing an intervention without thought for context is like baking a cake without thinking about the expertise of the baker, how long it needs to be in the oven and at what temperature, or whether the oven is functioning properly. We have emphasised the importance of context and systems in shaping the effectiveness of your intervention. These will shape the effectiveness of your intervention, much the same as the conditions within an oven will determine whether your cake is cooked to perfection or burnt to a crisp.

REAL-WORLD EXAMPLE: STAND UP FOR HEALTH

Sedentary behaviour can lead to a range of negative health outcomes. The workforce in contact (call) centres spend up to 95% of their day sitting. The aim of this project was to develop a *programme* theory for an intervention to reduce sedentary behaviour in contact centres. To maximise effectiveness and sustainability, such interventions need to be adaptive and take account of the local context, workplace culture and system into which the intervention is implemented.

Stakeholders were from the Ipsos MORI contact centre in Edinburgh, Scotland. The call centre had approximately 600 staff members, ranging in age from 18 to 65. The stakeholders included all types of staff (admin, call handlers, supervisors and managers). The national organisation (based in London) was also kept informed and updated. Based on a literature review and consultation with the stakeholder, modifiable and non-modifiable factors leading to sedentary behaviour in the contact centre were identified and presented in a fishbone diagram (see Figure 5.6).

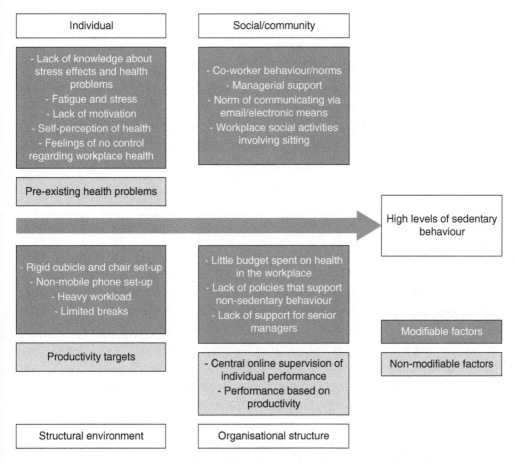

Figure 5.6   Fishbone diagram of modifiable and non-modifiable factors (Stand Up For Health)

Individual

Modifiable factors include knowledge of the health risks of sedentary behaviour, motivation and control over health within the workplace.

Social/community

Workplace norms and co-worker behaviour were significant modifiable factors. Additionally, the culture within the workplace around taking breaks was seen as another major factor.

Structural

The norm of seated, desk-based working is seen as a factor which could be easily modified by the researchers through the provision of various activities for which the researchers would help the centre to develop.

Organisational

Within the centre, few funds were put towards ergonomic support. However, the team conducting the intervention saw this as an opportunity to evidence the benefits of such items and thus labelled it as a modifiable factor. Additionally, a lack of structure for workplace activities was considered modifiable.

The team decided to target all the modifiable factors as they were all linked very much to each other and they had sufficient resources and assets within the call centre. For example, staff were keen, they had sufficient space and there were enough human resources to implement the intervention.

SUMMARY

This chapter has described the process involved in deciding which factors to target for intervention. This is the first step towards specifying how you will create change and is a fundamental step of the intervention development process. Some causal factors are more amenable to change (modifiable factors) than others (hard to modify), whereas some may lay beyond your reach in terms of available access and resources (non-modifiable). Whether a factor is modifiable, hard to modify or non-modifiable is highly dependent on context. In other words, what is modifiable to one team may be non-modifiable or hard to modify for another.

When choosing which factors to target, the following points should be considered:

1. Some factors contribute more to the problem than others. The contribution of factors can be identified through stakeholders in addition to research evidence and any available local data.
2. Factors exist within systems and as such relate to one other. You cannot understand any factor in isolation. It is often possible that the direct targeting of some factors may result in indirect knock-on effects on others. It is therefore important to create a theory of causes using a causal loop diagram. This will display how factors are related to one another and help you to select your targets based upon this.
3. The factors you decide to target should be guided by your available resources. Choose wisely, based on what is available to you in terms of both tangible and non-tangible resources.
4. Some factors may introduce ethical concerns if these are chosen as targets. What will the ethical implications be, if any? What boundaries will you create to ensure that your intervention stays within ethical standards and is acceptable?
5. It is important to keep in mind the three major pitfalls that may occur: focusing solely on factors at the individual level, focusing on increasing awareness and education only, and focusing on behaviours without paying attention to the context in which they occur. You can then begin to think about exactly how you intend to create change through targeting the variables selected.

FURTHER READING

Frieden, T. R. (2010) 'A framework for public health action: The Health Impact Pyramid', *American Journal of Public Health*, 100 (4): 590–5.

Komro, K. A. (2018) '25 years of complex intervention trials: reflections on lived and scientific experiences', *Research on Social Work Practice*, 28 (5): 523–31.

REFERENCES

Frieden, T. R. (2010) 'A framework for public health action: The Health Impact Pyramid', *American Journal of Public Health*, 100 (4): 590–5.

Gardner, B., Davies, A., and McAteer, J. (2010) 'Beliefs underlying UK parents' views towards MMR promotion interventions: a qualitative study', *Psychology, Health and Medicine*, 15 (2): 220–30.

Gubbels, J., van der Put, C., and Assink, M. (2019) 'Risk factors for school absenteeism and dropout: a meta-analytic review', *Journal of Youth and Adolescence*, 48 (9): 1637–67.

Hillsdon, M., Thorgood, M., White, I., and Foster, C. (2002) 'Advising people to take more exercise is ineffective: a randomized controlled trial of physical activity promotion in primary care', *International Journal of Epidemiology*, 31 (4): 808–15.

Komro, K. A. (2018) '25 years of complex intervention trials: reflections on lived and scientific experiences', *Research on Social Work Practice*, 28 (5): 523–31.

ACTIVITY ANSWERS

Scenario 5.1: Sleep problems

The factors listed as modifiable could be changed with relative ease. Bella could cut out coffee and wine before bed, reduce her screen time both before and in bed, and stop using her laptop in bed at night.

The hard to modify factors vary in terms of how much control she has over these, therefore some might be easier to change than others. For example, she could purchase a fan to lessen the heat from the heatwave, chat to her neighbours about the noise (she decides that purchasing earplugs is out of the question, since she needs to hear her daughter during the night) and speak with her boss about her feelings of workplace stress. The latter factor may be more difficult to change than the former factors, since change here would depend on an external influence – how amenable her boss is to modifying her workload and whether there is scope to do so.

Finally, she rules out tackling the following non-modifiable factors: her 8-month-old daughter who is teething and crying during the night, and her partner who has to work away. There is nothing she can do about these for the foreseeable future.

Bella decides that she will drink her last coffee of the day before 2pm and stop drinking alcohol on weeknights. She tries this for two weeks and notices some improvement but not much. She realises that, due to the complexity of the issue (represented by the number of factors contributing to her sleep problem), she must change more than one factor. Additionally, not all factors contribute equally to the problem. The consumption of coffee before bed, for example, is less of a factor than the baby crying for two hours at night. She decides that, in addition to making changes to her coffee and wine consumption, she will have a friendly talk with her neighbours about noise, and stop working on her laptop and using her phone in bed. Two weeks later, her sleeping has improved ... and her baby has a new tooth.

Activity 5.1: Reflection

The goal here is to encourage you to think about the nature of causal factors. Depending on the problem you identified, you should have compiled a list of modifiable, hard to modify and non-modifiable factors. You should also have thought through which of these factors might have the biggest impact on the problem if it were intervened upon. It is possible that the factors which have the biggest impact on the problem may be non-modifiable or hard to modify.

Activity 5.2: Decision making

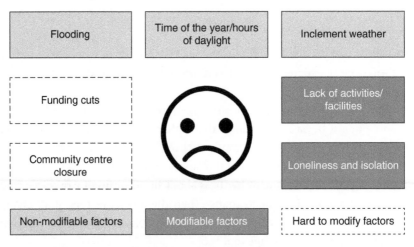

Figure 5.7   Modifiable, non-modifiable and hard to modify factors influencing low mood (Activity 5.2 answer)

Figure 5.7 shows a suggested answer. Lewis's team identifies three non-modifiable factors that are outside of his control: recent floods, darker evenings due to the time of year and inclement weather. The team categorises funding cuts and the recent community centre closure as hard to modify. In theory, these could be modified by re-establishing funding and reopening the community centre, but it is hard to see how Lewis could accomplish this in his position within the community centre and his current stakeholder group. He is working with a member of the local council, but this is a junior member of staff with little input in such decisions. Lewis identifies two factors as modifiable: lack of activities/facilities and loneliness and isolation. These are factors that he could work to change at two levels of intervention (the individual and community levels).

Activity 5.3: Planning

Who to invite and why: Jan invites her team and wider stakeholders. These individuals are invited because of their varied knowledge and experience, such as the team members in Scenario 5.2. Each participant will bring a different perspective to the workshop. Some of them represent the systems within which the intervention will be implemented, for instance the education system.

Factors for consideration based on information presented in the scenario

Potential factors for consideration include in-school and online bullying, substance use and a poor learning experience amongst pupils. The workshop should aim to identify any other potential factors before attempting to prioritise these.

Activities for use to reach consensus

Essentially, Jan's team needs to generate discussion, followed by some sort of voting exercise to reach agreement as a group. This process could follow the practical prioritisation exercise included in this chapter or variations of this. For example, you could split participants into small groups and ask them to produce a rich picture to illustrate the importance of each factor in contributing to the problem. This could then be followed by discussion and voting (e.g. using stickies or raised hands).

Knowledge link: This topic is also covered in Chapter 4

6

6SQUID STEP 3: IDENTIFYING HOW TO BRING ABOUT CHANGE – THEORY OF CHANGE

Learning objectives

After reading this chapter, you will be able to:

- Understand the role of theory in complex public health interventions
- Understand what a logic model is
- Understand what a theory of change is
- Develop a theory of change for use in intervention development.

Scenario 6.1

Antisocial behaviour in the community

Jeffrey is a police community liaison officer who has been asked to develop an intervention to reduce antisocial behaviour in the local community. He has formed a team consisting of local stakeholders, including representatives of a local community youth group, residents and a member of the local council. Residents have complained about antisocial behaviour, specifically groups of young people consuming alcohol at the local park. The team identifies seven potentially causal factors, shown in Figure 6.1.

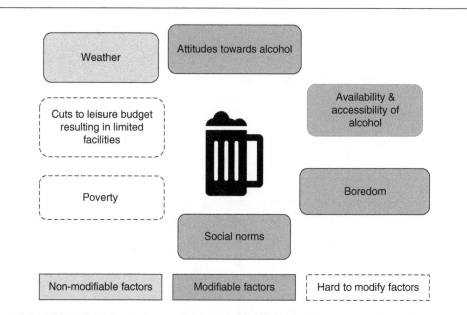

Figure 6.1 Modifiable, non-modifiable and hard to modify factors influencing antisocial behaviour

The problem seems to be worse during the summer months, likely due to the warm weather and tendency for people to stay outdoors for longer. This is a non-modifiable factor (the team cannot change the weather, as much as it might like to). Additionally, high levels of poverty in the area and cuts to the local authority leisure budget are likely causal factors. These are hard to modify since the team has little control over these. Four modifiable factors are identified:

1. Social norms (collective standards of behaviour, based on widely held beliefs, e.g. drinking alcohol makes you more fun amongst friends)
2. Attitudes towards alcohol
3. Availability and accessibility of alcohol; and
4. Boredom.

Activity 6.1

Decision making

For each of the four modifiable factors outlined in the opening scenario, the team must think about how to create change. For example, to change social norms, they think that raising awareness of alternative ways of thinking about alcohol will reduce favourable

(Continued)

views on alcohol and, in turn, reduce alcohol misuse. In your opinion, how might they go about creating change in the following modifiable factors:

1.   Availability and accessibility of alcohol?
2.   Boredom?
3.   Attitudes towards alcohol?

INTRODUCTION

A **theory** is a 'set of statements that organizes, predicts and explains observations; describing how phenomena relate to each other' (Bem and Looren de Jong, 1997: 5). Theory is part of our day-to-day lives. We use theory to help us navigate simple or complex choices on a day-to-day basis, from deciding how to prepare for a job interview, through what ingredients or meals to buy in the supermarket, to how to travel to work.

Imagine that you have an important job interview coming up. You must decide how best to present yourself. You can think of many ideas that might increase the likelihood of successfully securing the position. These ideas may involve how you dress, the cadence and tone of your voice, a firm handshake and making sufficient eye contact with the interviewer. As you think through how best to present yourself, what you are doing is theory-building. In other words, you are pulling together ideas that you believe are linked to successful job interviews. If you were to visualise your thinking, it might look something like the diagram shown in Figure 6.2. This process of theory-building – bringing ideas into focus, describing how they relate to one another and stating them clearly – is one of the most valuable tools at your disposal for intervention development.

The theory in Figure 6.2 consists of four statements and five constructs (component parts of theories). It states that 'dressing smartly' increases the likelihood of having a 'successful job interview' alongside similar statements for 'cadence and tone of voice',

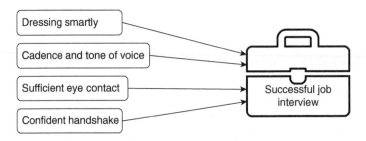

Figure 6.2   Simplified theory of job interview success

'sufficient eye contact' and a 'confident handshake'. This theory predicts and explains the outcome of a successful job interview by informing us of the influencing factors. Many frameworks for intervention development – including 6SQuID – incorporate use of theory as a central step in the intervention development process. Evidence suggests that interventions underpinned by theory are more likely to be effective compared to those that are not (Avery et al., 2013; Protogerou and Johnson, 2014). Not all theories are equal, however, and all should be viewed through the lens of evidence and context when thinking about their application. We should ask ourselves: Where did these ideas come from? Are they supported by any evidence? Do they apply to my circumstances? If we are aware of evidence demonstrating that the factors in our example can indeed influence the outcome of a job interview, we can say that our theory is evidence-based. However, can we be sure that the theory applies equally across circumstances and contexts? It is entirely possible that dressing smartly for an interview may not play as much of a role in helping you get the job in a company with a casual dress code. You might therefore have to tweak your theory to give yourself the best chance of success given your circumstances.

PROGRAMME THEORY IN PUBLIC HEALTH

Programme theory is a theory of how an intervention is expected to trigger a chain of outcomes through specified activities. Programme theory is comprised of two components: a theory of change and a theory of action. **Theory of change** specifies the mechanisms by which change is expected to occur. **Theory of action** explains how an intervention is constructed to activate your theory of change.

Knowledge link: This topic is also covered in Chapter 7

It is important to distinguish between theories of change and action and the roles they perform: the mechanism by which you intend to create change (theory of change) and how you intend to deliver or implement that change (theory of action). By developing your theory of change, you will describe the process by which you expect change will come about, for instance increasing the availability of fresh fruit and vegetables to improve nutrition in disadvantaged communities, rather than getting into the practical specifics of what the change will look like in your context, such as two deliveries of fresh fruit and vegetables twice a week to the local food bank (theory of action). This chapter focuses on describing the steps you should undertake to develop a theory of change. The approach we describe builds on that initially proposed by Weiss (1995).

Theories of change are not always successful, and a paper by Maini et al. (2018) provides a useful overview of how to, and how not to, develop a theory of change. Specifically, the authors mention the need to take account of how the intervention may interact within the wider system.

Specifying your short-, medium- and long-term outcomes

At the heart of programme theory is a chain of outcomes. This outcome chain is central to both theory of change and theory of action. It displays hypothesized cause and effect relationships between short-, medium- and long-term outcomes, which should be specified for each modifiable factor you have selected to target. Diagrams showing outcome chains are referred to as **logic models**. There are many types of logic models, and some have been developed to take account of the dynamics of complicated interventions. For a more detailed account of the range of logic models, see Mills et al. (2019).

Take, for example, the problem of healthcare-associated infections. These are infections that are acquired by patients in healthcare settings, having huge health and economic consequences. For example, data from the UK in 2016/17 show that such infections led to 22,800 patient deaths and cost the NHS £2.1 billion (Guest et al., 2020). Handwashing is the single most effective means of reducing healthcare-associated infections. There are a huge number of multi-level factors influencing this behaviour, but for the sake of simplicity, we have chosen to focus only on one: perceived behavioural control. This refers to individual perceptions of their ability to perform a behaviour. As an intervention developer, you might choose to target perceived behavioural control alongside other factors to increase handwashing behaviour. A simple logic model might therefore look like that shown in Figure 6.3.

For intervention development, this theory is only somewhat helpful in its current state. We can see that if we increase perceived behavioural control, we will likely increase handwashing and in the long term have an impact on levels of healthcare-associated infection. It is missing the lever by which to trigger this sequence of outcomes. This is sometimes referred to as the **change mechanism**. Complex interventions can have multiple change mechanisms at multiple levels. Your theory of change is essentially a specification of these change mechanisms and how they are expected to influence your short-, medium- and long-term outcomes.

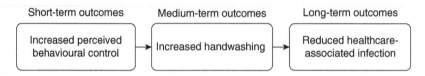

Figure 6.3 Simple logic model

HOW TO DEVELOP THEORY OF CHANGE

Developing theory of change involves both consideration of scientific theory and evidence, and working theory.

Scientific theory and evidence

Science by its nature involves theory-building – explaining how phenomena relate to one another – and rigorous testing to either confirm or refute hypotheses. In public health science, theories exist across political science, anthropology, medicine, social work, education, nursing, psychology, health geography and epidemiology. The multidisciplinary nature of public health has resulted in a huge number of theories, some of which purport to explain the same phenomena. For example, a scoping review identified 82 theories of behaviour and behaviour change across psychology, sociology, anthropology and economics alone (Davis et al., 2015). To further complicate matters, many scientific theories use the same constructs, albeit referring to them by different terms. For example, 'control' is a construct used across many behavioural theories. A review by Skinner (1996) identified over 100 conceptualisations of the 'control' construct across different theories, for example 'self-efficacy' within Social Cognitive Theory and 'perceived behavioural control' within the Theory of Planned Behaviour. Scientific theory in public health is therefore a messy business, and one that can be challenging – but not impossible – to navigate.

Scientific theories used in health intervention development

These are some of the more common theories used in the development of public health interventions, but this is by no means an exhaustive list.

Socio-ecological model

The socio-ecological model expresses health as a function of individuals and of the environment in which the individual lives – including family, social networks, organisations, communities and societies (Bronfenbrenner, 1977) (Figure 6.4). The individual is influenced by these external systems and he/she can in turn influence these systems directly or through groups and organisations. This approach underpins 6SQuID and our emphasis on a consideration of multiple levels of influence in order to understand and change complex public health problems.

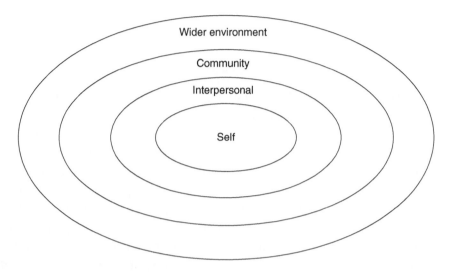

Figure 6.4 Socio-ecological model

Theory of planned behaviour (TPB)

The TPB states that behaviour is influenced by three constructs (Ajzen, 1991) (Figure 6.5). These are:

- attitude (positive or negative evaluation of a behaviour)
- subjective norm (social pressure to perform or not to perform a behaviour)
- perceived behavioural control (the perceived ease with which one can perform a behaviour).

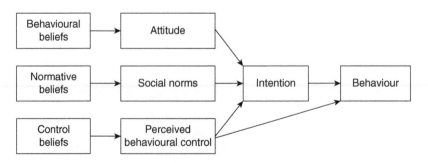

Figure 6.5 Theory of planned behaviour

These constructs are influenced by a further set of constructs. Attitudes are influenced by behavioural beliefs (beliefs about the outcomes of performing a behaviour). Subjective norms are influenced by normative beliefs (beliefs about social expectations in regard to the behaviour). Perceived behavioural control is influenced by control beliefs (beliefs about the presence of factors that may obstruct performance of the behaviour). The combined weight of attitude, subjective norm and perceived behavioural control forms a behavioural intention. Intention is considered to be the immediate antecedent to behaviour – in addition to perceived behavioural control. The TPB has been drawn upon to explain a variety of behaviours, including smoking, healthy eating, physical activity and sexual behaviour.

Operant learning theory

Operant learning theory describes the process underlying behaviour by reference to antecedents and consequences of that behaviour (Wong, 2008) (Figure 6.6). It posits that the antecedents of behaviour are either internal or external, for instance thoughts and environmental cues respectively. Behaviour is followed by consequences: rewards, withdrawal of rewards, punishment or escape (i.e. avoidance of punishment). The process underlying behaviour is described as a feedback loop in which behaviour (e.g. hand-hygiene behaviour) leads to consequences (e.g. infection), which feeds back into antecedents (internal: If I don't clean my hands in the future, I may catch another infection; or external: specific environments in which the threat of infection is present) and then back to behaviour. Operant learning theory has been applied to a number of problems, such as antibiotic prescribing and classroom management.

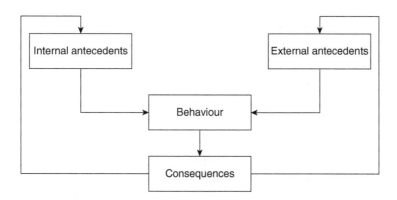

Figure 6.6   Operant learning theory

Self-efficacy theory of motivation

The self-efficacy theory of motivation states that previous experience, vicarious experience (e.g. experiences lived through others), social persuasion and physiological feedback (i.e. how experiences make you feel) impact upon self-efficacy (i.e. belief in your ability to succeed) which in turn impacts upon behaviour and performance (Bandura, 1977). This is shown in Figure 6.7.

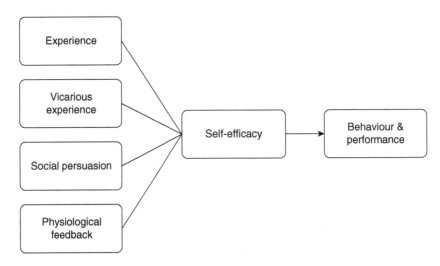

Figure 6.7   Self-efficacy theory of motivation

Transtheoretical model

The transtheoretical model views behaviour change as occurring in six stages (Prochaska and DiClemente, 1983) (Figure 6.8). The first stage is one of precontemplation in which the individual is unaware that their behaviour is problematic and needs to be changed. This is followed by the stage of contemplation, in which the individual intends to make changes to their behaviour in the future. Once the individual reaches the preparation stage, they are ready to take action and may take some small steps to changing their behaviour alongside developing the belief that changing their behaviour will lead to positive outcomes. At the action stage, the individual has recently changed his or her behaviour. This is followed by the maintenance and relapse prevention phase, during which the individual maintains the behaviour changes. Finally, the termination stage refers to the point at which an individual is certain they will no longer relapse into previously unhealthy behaviours.

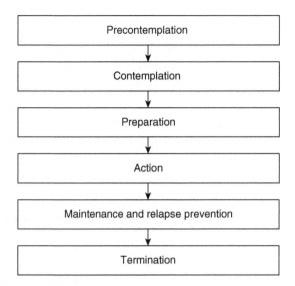

Figure 6.8 Transtheoretical model

Social-cognitive theory

Social-cognitive theory suggests that a behaviour is more likely to occur if people believe they have control over the outcome, there are few external barriers to performing the behaviour and when they have confidence in their ability to perform the behaviour (i.e. self-efficacy) (Bandura, 1986). This is shown in Figure 6.9.

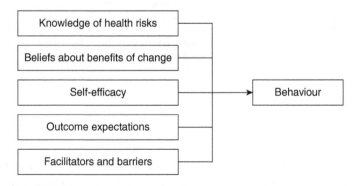

Figure 6.9 Social-cognitive theory

Nudge theory

Nudge theory assumes that individuals make most decisions subconsciously and this is influenced by contextual cues, and thus their behaviour can be manipulated by changing the way that choices are presented to them (Thaler and Sunstein, 2008) (Figure 6.10). By capitalising on the human subconscious, nudge ensures that the individual is unaware that their thoughts, decisions and behaviour are being influenced externally by what is referred to as choice architecture. Nudge operates on the view that it is legitimate to influence people's behaviour to make their lives healthier in a manner that neither is obtrusive nor entails compulsion. Proponents believe that nudge towards a positive behaviour may be effective and less prone to resistance by the target group than direct enforcement. Nudge emphasises the role of social and physical environments in shaping our behaviour.

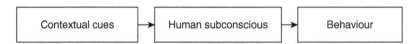

Figure 6.10   Nudge theory

Social norms theory

Social norms theory states that our behaviour is influenced by incorrect perceptions of how other members of our social groups think and act (Perkins and Berkowitz, 1986) (Figure 6.11). The theory states that overestimations of problem behaviour increase the occurrence of these behaviours, while underestimations of healthy behaviours discourage individuals from engaging in them.

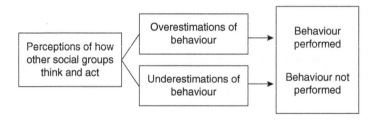

Figure 6.11   Social norms theory

Goal-setting theory

Goal-setting theory states that specific, attainable goals are more likely to lead to successful goal attainment (Locke and Latham, 1989) (Figure 6.12). This relationship is moderated by the level of commitment, the importance of the goal, self-efficacy, whether the individual receives performance feedback and the complexity of the task required to achieve the goal. The mechanisms underlying this relationship are whether the individual has a level of choice in selecting the goal, the effort applied, and the persistence and strategies for accomplishing the goal, such as planning.

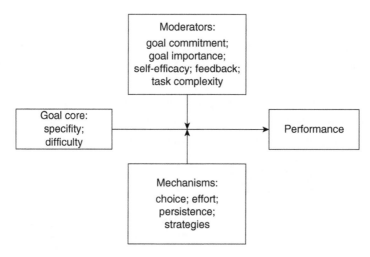

Figure 6.12 Goal-setting theory

Health belief model

The health belief model proposes that behaviour change occurs after an appraisal of perceived susceptibility (e.g. How likely am I to become unhealthy due to my eating habits?) and perceived severity (e.g. How severe do I think the impact could be?) (Rosenstock, 1974) (Figure 6.13). Taken together, these form a belief in a personal health threat. Additionally, appraisal occurs in terms of perceived benefits in engaging in more healthy behaviour (e.g. Am I likely to have more energy and feel lighter if I change my eating habits?) and perceived barriers (e.g. Do I have the money currently to buy more fruit and vegetables?). Taken together, these form a belief in the effectiveness of the health behaviour. Both belief in a personal health threat and belief in effectiveness of the health behaviour then determine whether that behaviour will occur.

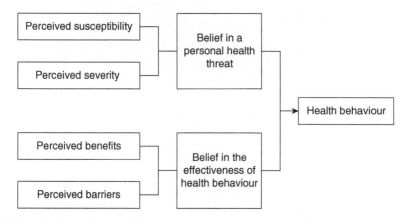

Figure 6.13 Health belief model

The COM-B model and behaviour change wheel

The COM-B model emphasises that behaviour is part of an interacting system of components consisting of capability, motivation and opportunity (Michie et al., 2011b) (Figure 6.14). The model proposes that individuals will engage in a behaviour if they have the capability to do so, feel sufficiently motivated to do so and have the opportunity to do so. The model forms the 'behaviour change wheel' around which are positioned nine intervention functions aimed at encouraging behaviour change (Figure 6.15). The outer rim of the wheel consists of various policy categories.

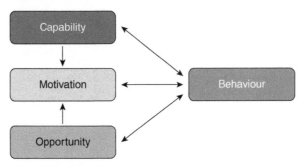

Figure 6.14   COM-B model

Source: Michie et al. (2011b) (CC BY)

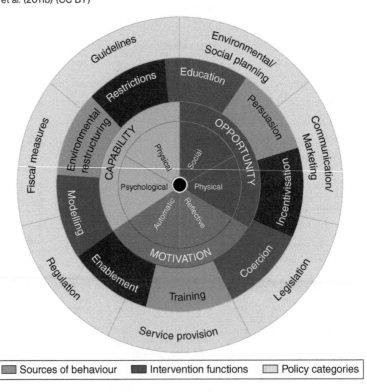

Figure 6.15   Behaviour change wheel

Source: Michie et al. (2011b) (CC BY)

HOW TO IDENTIFY RELEVANT SCIENTIFIC THEORIES

Literature searching is the best way to do this. If you have access to academic databases, a search of any given modifiable factor alongside the word theory or theories is likely to lead you to some potentially relevant theories. It is highly likely that someone may have already summarised the theoretical literature of relevance – in this case, it would usually be in the form of a theoretical review paper. We recognise that not everyone has access to academic search tools. In this case, we would advise broadly searching online as it is likely that you will find theory papers or broad theory overviews. Multiple theories may be of relevance.

In deciding on scientific theories to inform your intervention, you should consider:

- whether there is supporting evidence
- the need to draw on theory at more than one level of influence since the problem is complex
- the need to be flexible rather than rigid in your use of theory
- sustainability and the need to consider stakeholder views.

The need to consider supporting evidence

The first question that comes to mind when assessing the usefulness of a theory is usually: How good is it? How well does it explain the phenomena that it proclaims to and what is the evidence to support it? These are critical questions when deciding on how useful a theory is likely to be. Many of the theories outlined above have mixed explanatory value. The value of many of these theories has been the subject of debate after debate in the scientific literature for the past 20 years. For example, evidence suggests that the theory of planned behaviour predicts only around 20–30% of the variance in behaviour brought about by a TPB-based intervention (Armitage and Conner, 2001). Supporters of the theory have claimed that this may be due to methodological issues, primarily poor measurement of TPB constructs. However, given what we know about multilevel influences upon human behaviour in context, the issue may be far deeper than these methodological explanations. The TPB relies solely on individual-level constructs – beliefs, intentions and attitudes, and so on – to explain behaviour. We know that influences on behaviour are multilevel and embedded within systems. It is perhaps therefore not surprising that a theory consisting exclusively of individual-level constructs fails to account for greater than 20–30% of variance in behaviour.

Knowledge link: This topic is also covered in Chapter 2

The need to draw on theory at more than one level of influence

Many theories focus on one level of explanation, usually the individual, social or macro-environmental level. As explained elsewhere in this book, it is necessary, in public health intervention development, to consider multiple levels of influence. Doing so will increase the likelihood of your intervention having its intended effect. Public health and allied fields have seen a proliferation of psychological theories focused on explaining behaviour at the individual level. Unfortunately, the dominance of some scientific theories has arguably led to blinkered thinking with respect to attempts to improve public health outcomes. Whilst psychological theories are hugely relevant, it is unlikely that they will be useful alone in tackling complex public health problems, which requires a multilevel approach (Blue et al., 2014). It is important not to lose sight of the wider factors influencing behaviour, and to incorporate theory around these factors as part of your theory of change. In many cases, this consideration of wider factors will be incorporated via working theory which we will come onto in the next section.

Popular frameworks to assist intervention developers with theory selection have tended to focus primarily on behavioural theories (and in some cases, theories drawn from disciplines other than psychology) (Michie et al., 2011b). Supporters of this approach might argue that the reason such frameworks focus solely on behavioural theories is that these are the ones that are most well established. This is problematic. A well-established theory is not necessarily a good theory. For example, the usefulness of the TPB – a well-established theory spanning decades of research – has recently been the subject of fierce debate within the discipline of psychology itself (Sniehotta et al., 2014). Psychological science has some of the most well-established theories in the scientific literature, most of which have been around for many years. However, we should not lose sight of theoretical approaches from other disciplines, or younger theories, which may not be as well developed but still have something to tell us about the problems we are trying to tackle. Additionally, when established theories cannot account for the phenomena under investigation, we must not be scared to embark upon the development of new theoretical approaches. This is good science.

The need to be flexible rather than rigid in your use of theory

Many scientists align themselves with one particular theory. This can lead to inflexibility in terms of the extent to which a given theory can be adapted and modified. This theoretical purism results in a perspective in which one theory is understood to be the only theory of usefulness and relevance in regard to a specific phenomenon. The idea of using multiple theories or joining component parts of theories – constructs – is frowned upon by proponents of this approach. We argue that this use of multiple theories and joining of component parts is essential for good intervention development and is necessary due to the complexity of public health problems. This is something that intervention developers need to be comfortable with. It is entirely fine to use parts of theories rather than entire theories if that is more appropriate. It is not uncommon for academic colleagues to insist on the use of a specific scientific theory in the absence of contextual information. It is taken as a given that Theory X must apply if the phenomenon under investigation is the focus of that theory. This rigidity is unhelpful in the messy world of complex interventions and we would actively encourage you to be flexible in your approach.

It is also important to note that theories vary in terms of their specificity. For example, the socio-ecological model describes influences upon individuals, therefore by its nature is extremely broad. Contrast this with a theory like operant learning theory which is extremely specific, talking about the process underlying behaviour by reference to antecedents and consequences of behaviour. The usefulness of a theory is not determined by its level of specificity, but rather whether it is useful in the context in which it will be applied. For example, if you set out to develop an intervention to increase physical activity, you may choose to draw upon operant learning theory which would suggest that rewarding occurrences of physical activity is likely to reinforce that behaviour. However, as we know, behaviour occurs in context, therefore reliance solely upon operant learning theory and a mechanism of reward is unlikely to be effective in and of itself. Similarly, the socio-ecological model provides a useful framework for understanding the multilevel influences on individuals. However, the socio-ecological model is a universal theory which applies across the board. It does not, therefore, provide specific information about how to go about changing the modifiable factors which matter to your specific problem and context. This is perhaps a good place to reflect on what we stated earlier in the chapter: theory in public health can be a messy business.

Sustainability and the need to consider stakeholder views

As mentioned in Chapter 2, sustainability is an important component of any intervention, and it is often necessary and valuable to incorporate it into your theory of change. At this stage, it is useful to articulate what aspects of sustainability are important and how sustainability can be achieved by drawing on stakeholder views. For example, in a study of developing an intervention to increase physical activity in women who used Bingo Clubs (Well!Bingo) we identified the following aspects that were integral to sustainability:

- The women and the bingo club felt ownership of the problem and the solutions.
- Any interventions took account of the systems in which they were implemented (in this case the bingo club).
- Any intervention was linked to the culture of the organisation rather than competing with it (activities were fun and took place before or after the bingo sessions).
- There were the resources (and/or assets) needed to maintain the intervention after it had been developed and piloted (the bingo club provided a space for the activities as well as free refreshments).

We were then able to write several of these into our programme theory (see Figure 6.16).

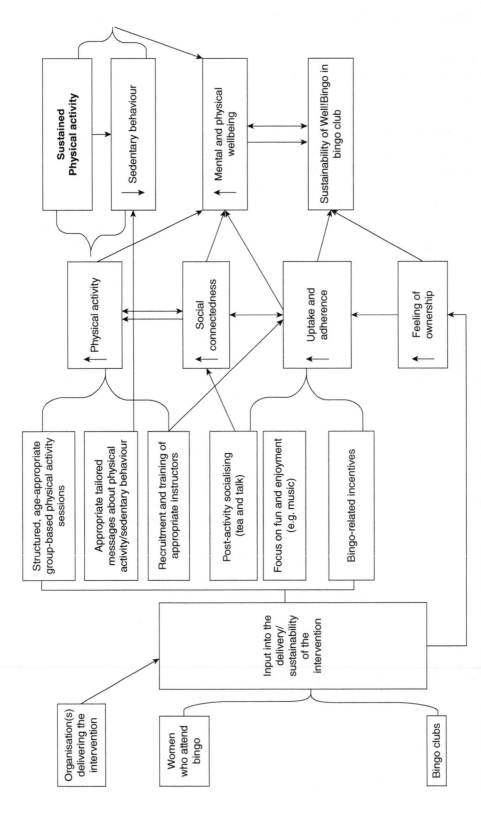

Figure 6.16 Incorporating sustainability into your theory of change: Well!Bingo

In the Stand Up For Health (SUH) intervention, a key factor for sustainability was the need for an organisational committee comprising of all levels of staff. They were responsible for developing activities and communications and ensuring that SUH remained on the workplace agenda. Another key factor was embedding it within the organisational culture, so that it became part of normal practice. For example, in one contact centre the focus on reducing sedentary behaviour was written into the induction packs for all new staff.

Mayne (2020) describes the COM-B model (presented in our list of scientific theories) as a useful framework for understanding sustainability in terms of interventions, stating that

- any opportunities (the outside factors that make the behaviour possible or prompt it) would need to continue to be available; and
- the motivation that brought about the change would also need to remain.

USING SCIENTIFIC THEORY

Let's revisit Jeffrey's team from our opening scenario. It identified four modifiable factors contributing to alcohol misuse in his community, one of which was social norms. In his logic model, the outcomes chain for this modifiable factor looks like that shown in Figure 6.17.

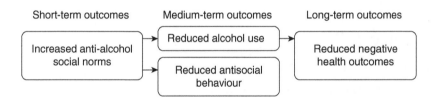

Figure 6.17 Outcomes chain

You can see that team members aim to increase anti-alcohol social norms in the short term. They hypothesise that this will lead to reduced alcohol use and reduced antisocial behaviour in the medium term. In the longer term, they hypothesise that reductions in alcohol use will lead to reduced negative health outcomes. They now need to identify the mechanism of change that will trigger these outcomes.

After searching for theories related to social norms, the team decides that social norms theory provides a useful theory to inform its change mechanism. Remember, the change mechanism is what triggers the outcome chain. The theory selected states that behaviour is influenced by incorrect perceptions of how other members of our social groups think and act. Overestimations of problem behaviour increase the occurrence of these behaviours, while underestimations of healthy behaviours discourage individuals from engaging in them. The team decides that its change mechanism will be to raise awareness of alternative ways of thinking about alcohol across the community. Social norms theory suggests that this will affect individual perceptions of how others think and act and likely lead to reductions in alcohol misuse. The team would need to check that this makes sense in terms of the local context (we come on to this in the next section). The team would then update its outcomes chain with the change mechanism to form a theory of change, as shown in Figure 6.18.

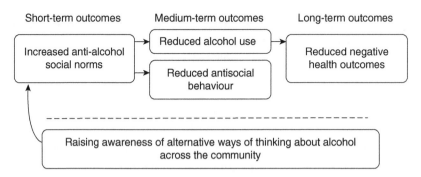

Figure 6.18 Theory of change (outcomes chain including mechanism of change for modifiable factor: social norms)

Activity 6.2

Decision making

Mo is part of a team that is developing an intervention to increase staff handwashing in hospital wards. They have identified factors influencing this behaviour, one of which is lack of motivation. Their outcome chain hypothesises that increased motivation will lead to increased handwashing and reduced healthcare-associated infection, as shown in Figure 6.9.

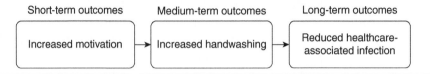

Figure 6.19 Outcomes chain for modifiable factor – motivation

The team has decided to use operant learning theory to inform its decision around how best to trigger this sequence of outcomes. Finish this theory of change by adding the change mechanism to the outcomes chain.

WORKING THEORY

Theories of change draw upon both scientific theory and working theory. **Working theory** can be defined as non-scientific stakeholder understanding of a phenomenon, drawing upon local and contextual knowledge and experience. Context is a key consideration – as emphasised in the opening scenario (and throughout this book) – when developing interventions to tackle complex public health problems. Context informs every decision made in the intervention development process. If it does not, then it is likely that you are doing it wrong.

Using working theory

Working theory is generated by talking to stakeholders. The reason we emphasise co-production and stakeholder involvement so much throughout this book is precisely because of the importance of information related to the context in which your intervention will be implemented. By failing to incorporate local and contextual knowledge and experiences, your intervention is likely to fail. By the time you reach this step, you will have formed a team consisting of relevant stakeholders. Your team should examine and discuss the proposed outcome chains, and any potentially relevant theories which could inform the change mechanisms to trigger these. Questions to ask include: 'Given your experience and understanding of the problem and context, what do you think would trigger these outcomes?', and 'Are the change mechanisms proposed by theory X, Y and Z likely to trigger these outcomes in this context?'. At this stage, you will need to consider how your proposed change mechanisms are likely to operate, given the systems in which you aim to deliver your intervention.

Knowledge link: This topic is also covered in Chapter 2

To illustrate this, in Scenario 6.1 one of the modifiable factors contributing to alcohol misuse is boredom. The team's outcome chain for this modifiable factor is shown in Figure 6.20. They propose that reducing boredom in the short term will lead to reduced alcohol use in the medium term and reduced negative health outcomes in the longer term. As a team, they discuss how best to trigger this outcomes chain. There is consensus amongst them that young people have little to do in the community, especially in the evenings and at weekends. They therefore agree that providing alternative or diversionary activities will trigger this outcomes chain. Jeffrey updates his outcomes chain to include this mechanism of change and now has a complete theory of change, as shown in Figure 6.21. He should also need to consider which systems may impact on these diversionary activities. Such activities may be delivered by the police, youth clubs, the third sector or community volunteers.

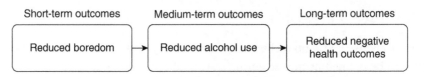

Figure 6.20   Outcomes chain for modifiable factor – boredom

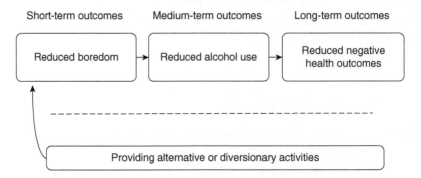

Figure 6.21   Theory of change (outcomes chain including mechanism of change for modifiable factor – boredom)

Whilst it is useful to develop working theory directly with your team, we would advise that you also consult with wider stakeholders through a workshop. You could conduct some interviews or focus groups, however we feel that a workshop format allows for more flexibility and creativity in terms of the methods employed. Such a workshop should be geared towards:

i.   presenting your outcome chains
ii.   generating suggested change mechanisms – how to trigger outcome chains – based on participants' contextual knowledge and experience
iii. presenting any change mechanisms sourced from scientific theory and discussion of their relevance to context
iv.   reaching consensus as to which should form your theory of change.

INTERVENTION DEVELOPMENT TOOL: BRAINSTORMING AND RANKING

Brainstorming and ranking can be useful for generating ideas and gaining a sense of their importance to workshop participants. In relation to generating working theory, this technique can be used to identify change mechanisms and the extent to which participants feel they are relevant to the local context within which the intervention will be implemented.

Suggested steps for this method are listed below. We encourage you to be creative and to adapt these steps as you wish:

1. Split participants into small groups.
2. Ask each group to discuss the presented outcome chains and to brainstorm the potential change mechanisms that are likely to trigger these, given their knowledge of context. Group members should write these on cards or Post-it notes.
3. After brainstorming, the lead facilitator should begin to collate the change mechanisms and group any that are similar at the front of the room. The facilitator should include any change mechanisms also identified via scientific theory. This should be followed by a group discussion in which the lead facilitator asks the group for their views on each change mechanism suggested.
4. The facilitator should ask members of the wider group to rank the suggested change mechanisms in terms of the extent to which they think these are likely to trigger outcome chains, given their knowledge of systems and context. This can be done using numbered stickies, with 1 being most likely to trigger an outcome chain.
5. The facilitator should present rankings, followed by discussion and any changes.
6. As it is likely you will have multiple outcome chains, you may need to conduct this exercise more than once.

THE IMPORTANCE OF ANTICIPATING UNINTENDED CONSEQUENCES

As an intervention developer, your goal is to create positive change. However, it is important to note that interventions can have both positive and negative consequences. There have been recent calls for more consideration to be given to potential unintended consequences resulting from intervention attempts (Bonell et al., 2015). You should therefore examine your theory of change to anticipate potential unintended outcomes which may arise as a consequence of intervening. For example, in providing alternative or diversionary activities to reduce alcohol use, it is possible that Jeffrey's team may inadvertently *facilitate* alcohol use by providing more opportunities for young people to mix (negative consequence) and/or contribute to the development of new skills and interests (positive consequence). It is essential to mitigate against any negative outcomes should they occur. For example, Jeffrey's team might consider increasing supervision at these activities to mitigate the likelihood of these facilitating alcohol use. He could add staffing capacity to the intervention if funds permit, so that more staff are present during the activities. Or he could reduce the number of young people at each activity, making sessions easier for fewer staff to supervise. Stakeholder input is again hugely important when considering unwanted outcomes and what can be done to mitigate against these, since stakeholders are far more likely to be able to anticipate these based on their experiential knowledge. You should build this issue into any engagement work – workshops and so on – at this stage, by including it as a topic for discussion.

REAL-WORLD EXAMPLE: STAND UP FOR HEALTH

The next section aims to consolidate your learning in this chapter, using an example of a real-world intervention to reduce sedentary behaviour in the workplace: Stand Up For Health. Sedentary behaviour can lead to a range of negative health outcomes. The workforce in contact (call) centres spend up to 95% of their day sitting. Stand Up For Health aimed to develop an intervention to reduce sedentary behaviour in this setting. To maximise effectiveness and sustainability, such interventions need to be adaptive and take account of the local context, workplace culture and system into which the intervention is implemented. Stakeholders were from the Ipsos MORI contact centre in Edinburgh, Scotland. Based on a literature review and consultation with the stakeholder, modifiable and non-modifiable factors leading to sedentary behaviour in the contact centre were identified and presented in a fishbone diagram, as shown in Figure 6.22.

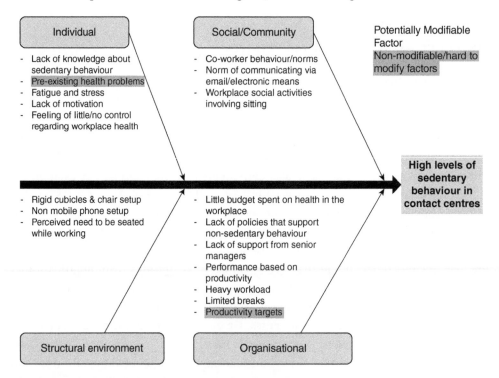

Figure 6.22   Stand Up For Health (fishbone diagram)

Individual

Modifiable factors include knowledge of the health risks of sedentary behaviour, motivation and control over health within the workplace.

Social/community

Workplace norms and co-worker behaviour were significant modifiable factors. Additionally, the culture within the workplace around taking breaks was seen as another major factor.

Structural

The norm of seated, desk-based working is seen as a factor which could be easily modified by the researchers through the provision of various activities for which the researchers would help the centre to develop.

Organisational

Within the centre, little funding was put towards ergonomic support. However, the researchers saw this as an opportunity to evidence the benefits of such items and thus labelled it as a modifiable factor. Additionally, a lack of structure for workplace activities was considered modifiable.

The researchers and stakeholders decided to target all the modifiable factors as they were all linked very much to each other and they had sufficient resources and assets within the call centre. For example, staff were keen, they had sufficient space and there were enough human resources to implement the intervention.

The team began to construct a programme theory, the specification of an outcomes chain being the first step towards accomplishing this. The outcomes chain is a roadmap of outcomes and how they relate to one another, as shown in Figure 6.23.

You can see here that changing the targeted modifiable factors is expected to lead to staff sitting less and moving more at work in the medium term. Note that the intervention developers have listed an unintended positive consequence which is that this change in behaviour might become habitual and extend to other circumstances – staff sitting less and moving more outside of work. In the longer term, a number of outcomes are listed in terms of benefits for staff and also benefits for the centre. For staff, these include improved fitness, better mental wellbeing and musculoskeletal health. For the centre, these include increased productivity, reduced absenteeism and a healthy, happier workplace.

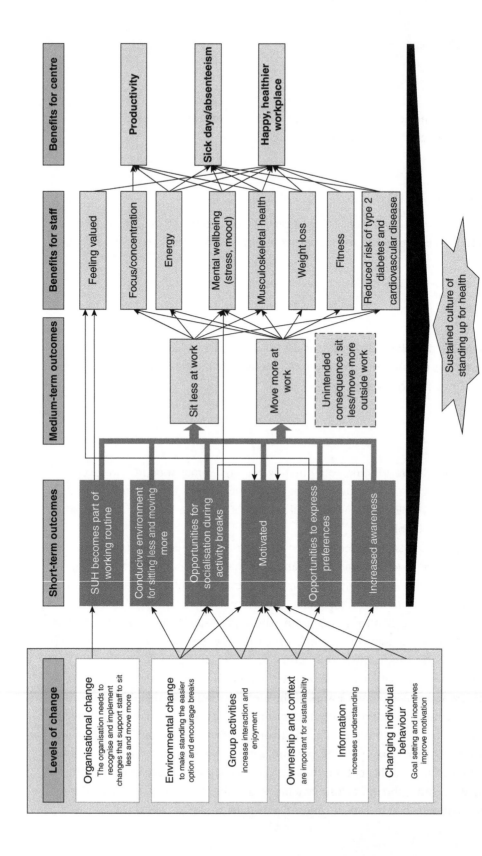

Figure 6.23 Stand Up For Health: theory of change (logic model with proposed change mechanisms)

Change mechanisms are listed to the left of Figure 6.23. Note that these are listed as occurring at different levels of change, from individual behaviour to organisational level change. These change mechanisms were identified through drawing upon a mixture of scientific theory and working theory. For example, intervention developers propose that goal-setting and the provision of incentives (the mechanism of change) will increase motivation, which will in turn lead to sitting less and moving more at work, which will in turn lead to a number of benefits for staff, including increased focus and concentration and fitness, in addition to wider benefits for the centre. The mechanism of change in this instance is informed by goal-setting theory and operant learning theory. Similarly, intervention developers propose that recognition and implementation of changes which support staff to sit less and move more will lead to Stand Up For Health becoming part of working routine. The intervention developers hypothesise that this will lead directly to staff feeling valued and a happier, healthier workplace in the longer term. It will also directly lead to staff sitting less and moving more at work and a number of long-term outcomes. The mechanism of change in this instance is informed by stakeholder views as to how best to trigger this outcomes chain, i.e. this was informed by working theory.

Activity 6.3

Reflection

Using the diagram outlined in Figure 6.23, specify the theories of change underpinning Stand Up For Health. In other words, specify the change mechanisms at each level and the pathways with which they are expected to impact on short-term, medium-term and long-term outcomes.

SUMMARY

This chapter described the role of theory in complex public health interventions. We introduced the concept of programme theory – theory describing how your intervention will contribute to a chain of outcomes. Programme theory is comprised of theory of change and theory of action. Theory of change is the mechanism by which change comes about, whereas theory of action describes the specific strategies you will use to activate your theory of change. Outcome chains – otherwise known as logic models – can be used to display hypothesized cause and effect relationships between short-, medium- and long-term outcomes, and we recommend that you begin to construct one of these to clearly begin to demonstrate your programme theory. It is essential to specify your mechanisms for creating change in relation to your modifiable factors and to clearly illustrate the pathway by which this change will impact on the problem you have chosen to tackle. These mechanisms of change will trigger the outcome chains within your logic model, and therefore make up your theory of change. However, you must be mindful of the potential for unplanned outcomes resulting from your intervention. These should be anticipated and mitigated against. The next chapter will describe the process of developing your theory of action, i.e. activities that will activate your theory of change.

FURTHER READING

Blue, S., Shove, E., Carmona, C., and Kelly, M. P. (2014) 'Theories of practice and public health: understanding (unhealthy) practices', *Critical Public Health*, 26: 36–50.

Bruer, E., Lee, L., de Silva, M., and Lund, C. (2015) 'Using theory of change to design and evaluate public health interventions: a systematic review', *Implementation Science*, 11: 63.

Davis, R., Campbell, R., Hildon, Z., Hobbs, L., and Michie, S. (2015) 'Theories of behaviour and behaviour change across the social and behavioural sciences: a scoping review', *Health Psychology Review*, 9 (3): 323–44.

Maini, R., Mounier-Jack, S., and Borghi, J. (2018) 'How to and how not to develop a theory of change to evaluate a complex intervention: reflections on an experience in the Democratic Republic of Congo', *BMJ Global Health*, 3: e000617.

Mayne, J. (2020) 'Sustainability analysis of intervention benefits: a theory of change approach', *Canadian Journal of Program Evaluation*, 35 (2): 204–21. doi:10.3138/cjpe.70004

Mills, T., Lawton, R., and Sheard, L. (2019) 'Advancing complexity science in healthcare research: the logic of logic models', *BMC Medical Research Methodology*, 19: 55. https://doi.org/10.1186/s12874-019-0701-4

REFERENCES

Ajzen, I. (1991) 'The theory of planned behavior', *Organizational Behavior and Human Decision Processes*, 50 (2): 179–211.

Armitage, C. J., and Conner, M. (2001) 'Efficacy of the theory of planned behaviour: a meta-analytic review', *British Journal of Social Psychology*, 40: 471–99.

Avery, K. N., Donovan, J. L., Horwood, J., and Lane, J. A. (2013) 'Behavior theory for dietary interventions for cancer prevention: a systematic review of utilization and effectiveness in creating behavior change', *Cancer Causes and Control*, 24: 409–20.

Bandura, A. (1977) 'Self-efficacy: toward a unifying theory of behavioral change', *Psychological Review*, 84: 191–215.

Bandura, A. (1986) *Social Foundations of Thought and Action: A Social Cognitive Theory.* Hoboken, NJ: Prentice-Hall.

Bem, S., and Looren de Jong, H. (1997) *Theoretical Issues in Psychology.* London: Sage.

Blue, S., Shove, E., Carmona, C., and Kelly, M. P. (2014) 'Theories of practice and public health: understanding (unhealthy) practices', *Critical Public Health, 26*: 36–50.

Bonell, C., Jamal, F., Melendez-Torres, G. J., and Cummins, S. (2015) '"Dark logic": theorising the harmful consequences of public health interventions', *Journal of Community and Epidemiological Health, 69*: 95–8.

Bronfenbrenner, U. (1977) 'Toward an experimental ecology of human development', *American Psychologist, 32*: 513–31.

Davis, R., Campbell, R., Hildon, Z., Hobbs, L., and Michie, S. (2015) 'Theories of behaviour and behaviour change across the social and behavioural sciences: a scoping review', *Health Psychology Review, 9* (3): 323–44.

Guest, J. F., Keating, T., Gould, D., and Wigglesworth, N. (2020) 'Modelling the annual NHS costs and outcomes attributable to healthcare-associated infections in England', *BMJ Open, 22*; *10*(1), doi: 10.1136/bmjopen-2019-033367

Locke, E., and Latham, G. P. (1989) *A Theory of Goal Setting and Task Performance*. Hoboken, NJ: Prentice-Hall.

Maini, R., Mounier-Jack, S., and Borghi, J. (2018) 'How to and how not to develop a theory of change to evaluate a complex intervention: reflections on an experience in the Democratic Republic of Congo', *BMJ Global Health*, 3: e000617.

Michie, S., Ashford, S., Sniehotta, F., Dombrowski, S., Bishop, A., and French, D. (2011a) 'A refined taxonomy of behaviour change techniques to help people change their physical activity and healthy eating behaviours: The CALO-RE taxonomy', *Psychology and Health, 26* (11): 1479–98.

Michie, S., van Stralen, M., and West, R. (2011b) 'The behaviour change wheel: a new method for characterising and designing behaviour change interventions', *Implementation Science, 6*: 42.

Mills, T., Lawton, R., and Sheard, L. (2019) 'Advancing complexity science in healthcare research: the logic of logic models', *BMC Medical Research Methodology, 19*: 55. https://doi.org/10.1186/s12874-019-0701-4

Perkins, H. W., and Berkowitz, A. (1986) 'Perceiving the community norms of alcohol use among students: some research implications for campus alcohol education programming', *International Journal of Addiction, 21*: 961–76.

Prochaska, J., and DiClemente, C. (1983) 'Stages and processes of self-change of smoking: toward an integrative model of change', *Journal of Consulting and Clinical Psychology, 51* (3): 390–5.

Protogerou, C., and Johnson, B. T. (2014) 'Factors underlying the success of behavioural HIV-prevention interventions for adolescents: a meta-review', *AIDS and Behaviour, 18*: 1847–63.

Rosenstock, I. M. (1974) 'The health belief model and preventive behaviour', *Health Education Monographs, 2* (4): 354–86.

Skinner, E. A. (1996) 'A guide to constructs of control', *Journal of Personality and Social Psychology, 71* (3): 549–70.

Sniehotta, F. F., Presseau, J., and Araujo-Soares, V. (2014) 'Time to retire the theory of planned behaviour', *Health Psychology Review, 8* (1): 1–7.

Thaler, R., and Sunstein, C. (2008) *Nudge: Improving Decisions about Health, Wealth, and Happiness*. New Haven, CT: Yale University Press.

Weiss, C. (1995) 'Nothing as practical as good theory: exploring theory-based evaluation for comprehensive community initiatives for children and families', in J. P. Connell (ed.),

New Approaches to Evaluating Community Initiatives: Concepts, Methods, and Contexts. Washington, DC: Aspen Institute, pp. 65–92.

Wong, S. E. (2008) 'Operant learning theory', in B. A. Thyer, K. M. Sowers and C. N. Dulmus (eds), *Comprehensive Handbook of Social Work and Social Welfare, vol. 2. Human Behavior in the Social Environment.* Hoboken, NJ: John Wiley & Sons, pp. 69–99.

ACTIVITY ANSWERS

Activity 6.1: Decision making

Availability and accessibility of alcohol:

- More frequent police contact with local supermarkets will reduce the likelihood of illegal sales.
- Providing education to local supermarkets will reduce the likelihood of illegal sales.

Boredom:

- Provision of tailored (to the interests of young people in the area) alternative diversionary activities will reduce boredom.
- Increasing access to sports at the weekends and in the evenings will reduce boredom.

Attitudes towards alcohol:

- Providing information about the health consequences of alcohol use will change attitudes.
- Changing social norms around alcohol will change attitudes.

Activity 6.2: Decision making

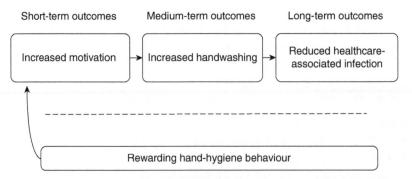

Figure 6.24 Proposed diagram outlining possible method for triggering increased motivation, handwashing and reduced healthcare-associated infections

The team could consider rewarding handwashing behaviour to increase motivation and trigger subsequent outcomes.

Activity 6.3: Reflection

Organisational change in the form of support from management will lead to the intervention becoming part of the working routine, which will have the effect of contributing to the success of the intervention. This will mean staff sitting less and moving more at work, followed by a range of benefits for staff and the call centre as a whole.

Environmental change is required to make standing the easier option and encourage breaks. This leads to a range of intermediate outcomes, including an environment conducive to sitting less and moving more and opportunities for socialisation during activity breaks. These lead to sitting less and moving more, which leads to an increase in short-term outcomes such as concentration, energy, mental wellbeing (from both the socialisation and the sitting less), fewer musculoskeletal issues, weight loss, fitness and a reduction in non-communicable diseases such as diabetes. This leads to greater productivity, reduced sick days and a healthier, happier workplace. In other words, benefits are seen for staff and the call centre as a whole.

Group activities increase interaction and enjoyment which lead to a motivation to sit less and move more and provide more opportunities for socialisation. The arrows in the diagram indicate that it is a loop – that the more motivated you are, the more likely you are to socialise and that in turn makes you more motivated. This leads to sitting less and moving more, in addition to benefits for staff and the call centre as a whole.

Ownership is important for sustainability – opportunities to express preferences lead to increased motivation and a feeling of being valued, which in turn lead to benefits for staff and the call centre as a whole.

Information increases understanding which leads to an increased awareness of the risks of sedentary behaviour, and increased motivation to take part in activities which in turn lead to the other outcomes.

Individual behaviour change through goal setting and incentives will lead to increased motivation. This will result in staff sitting less and moving more at work, followed by benefits for staff and for the call centre as a whole.

7

6SQUID STEP 4: IDENTIFYING HOW TO DELIVER CHANGE MECHANISMS – THEORY OF ACTION

Learning objectives

By the end of this chapter, you will be able to:

- Define theory of action
- Optimise delivery of your change mechanisms
- Develop a theory of action for use in intervention development.

INTRODUCTION

Knowledge link: This topic is also covered in Chapter 6

The previous chapter described how to develop a **theory of change** by specifying an outcomes chain and identifying change mechanisms either through reviewing the scientific literature, consulting with stakeholders or a mixture of both. This chapter describes how to develop a **theory of action**, i.e. how to construct an intervention that will activate your underpinning theory of change. Your underpinning theory of change and activating theory of action make up your intervention's **programme theory**. To clearly illustrate how to go about developing a theory of action, we will spend the majority of this chapter applying the recommended steps to what is possibly one of the biggest public health interventions of modern times: the response to COVID-19. First, it is necessary to ensure that you have a clear understanding of the distinction and relationship between theories of change and theories of action.

UNDERSTANDING THE RELATIONSHIP BETWEEN THEORY OF CHANGE AND THEORY OF ACTION

Theory of change and theory of action essentially explain the same thing but at different levels of explanation. Theory of change requires identifying your change mechanisms and how you expect them to influence your outcomes. Theory of action requires identifying and planning how you will activate these change mechanisms in practice. Theory of change is more abstract whereas theory of action is more concrete and operates at the local level. Both are complementary, together comprising the programme theory.

Knowledge link: This topic is also covered in Chapter 6

A theory of change is like a row of interconnected containers that must be filled to a certain level before they trigger a response in each other. Theory of change links an outcomes chain and the mechanism that is required to trigger it. In this sense, theories of change are abstract theories. Your theory of action, on the other hand, is less abstract and more concrete. It is whatever is poured into the containers to activate the theory of change, including the type of item that is poured (water, beads, feathers), which we refer to as format the rate at which they are poured (quickly, slowly, etc.) and how often they are poured (once, twice or three times a week or an hour, etc.). In other words, your theory of action is the specific ingredients that make up your intervention. To activate your theory of change, the ingredients must be delivered at the correct 'dose'. However, unlike medicinal interventions, the precise ingredients which make up this dose may change depending on the context in which the intervention is being delivered. Essentially, theory of action operationalises your theory of change in such a way that it activates it.

Take the example of an intervention to tackle the problem of poor nutrition. A possible theory of change may be that increasing the availability of healthy foods (mechanism) will result in people eating more healthy foods (short-term outcome), improving their nutritional intake (medium-term outcome) and better overall health (long-term outcome). You can see here that this is quite abstract in that it does not go into the specifics of delivery. It specifies only the relationship between the mechanism of change (informed by evidence and stakeholder consultation) and short-, medium- and long-term outcomes (remember, we refer to this as an outcomes chain). The specification of how this theory of change will be applied in a specific context is a theory of action. How it is applied will differ, depending on contextual factors and the assets available to those implementing the intervention. In the UK,

Knowledge link: This topic is also covered in Chapter 6

the intervention developer might decide to seek sponsorship and work with large super-markets to make healthy food available weekly in community locations such as the local library. Implementing this intervention in rural India would require a different approach. In short, the theory of change remains unchanged. The way it is activated – the theory of action – can change.

You may wonder why these two levels of explanation are necessary. To be explicit, the theory of change describes the rationale linking your mechanism of change to a chain of outcomes. This can be taken and applied elsewhere, i.e. it can inform the development of theories of action (which are context-dependent). Indeed, the theory of action describes how the theory of change will be activated in a specific context. It represents the nuts and bolts of your intervention. The theory of action cannot be taken and applied elsewhere without proper consideration as to whether the activities outlined are likely to work in another setting. In many cases, a different theory of action may be required to activate the same underpinning theory of change.

As this book was being written, COVID-19 was declared a pandemic by the World Health Organisation. The world began to see an increase in community spread of the virus, with a resultant increase in numbers of hospitalisations and deaths across the world, and social and economic consequences. This upsurge in community transmission was fol-lowed by public health interventions on a scale never seen before in our lifetime. These interventions often shared the same underpinning theories of change but were delivered differently – the activating theories of action – depending on the local, national and inter-national contexts in which they were applied. We have therefore chosen to devote a large section of this chapter to this problem, to illustrate how to develop a theory of action. We will also use this as an opportunity to consolidate our learning from Chapter 6, since theory of change and theory of action are closely interlinked.

To specify how your programme will be constructed, you must first understand the mechanisms by which you intend to trigger your outcome chain, i.e. your theories of change. This is where we will begin.

THE PROBLEM OF COVID-19: POTENTIAL THEORIES OF CHANGE

Figure 7.1 shows theories of change aimed at tackling the problem of COVID-19 and how these relate to intended outcomes. Note the change mechanisms. These are the triggers by which to activate the specified outcomes chain, which contains short-, medium- and long-term outcomes. Also note that these are multilevel, from population level (legisla-tion) to individual level (education and practical guidance). Intervening solely at a single level is unlikely to be as effective as intervening at multiple levels when it comes to public health problems, as we have emphasised throughout this book.

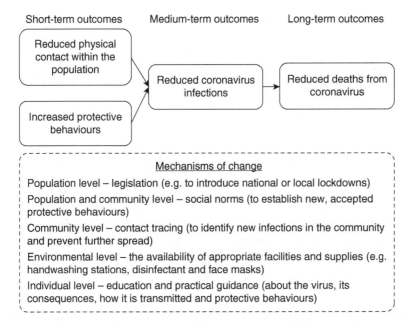

Figure 7.1   Theories of change geared towards tackling the problem of COVID-19

To activate this theory of change, the change mechanisms must be delivered at the correct 'dose', much of which is highly context dependent. You can see from this example that the theory of change is *context independent* – it is not referencing a specific context or getting into the nuts and bolts of implementation. For example, the theory of change proposes that the introduction of legislation will reduce physical contact within the population and increase protective behaviours, reducing new infections and subsequent deaths. How this is applied in practice (the theory of action) may differ based on the context in which you are implementing your intervention. For example, one country might decide to allow physical contact at certain times of the day but impose a curfew in the evening, whilst another might decide to advise against physical contact at all times of the day except for essential purposes. Your theory of action will therefore specify the 'dose' at which your intervention will be delivered, given the context it will be applied in, and the systems where the activities will take place.

DEVELOPING A THEORY OF ACTION

The operationalisation of change mechanisms is at the core of theory of action. This is highly dependent on the context in which you intend to implement your intervention. **Operationalisation** refers to the practical specification of activities employed to activate your underpinning theory of change. Theory of action is essentially the operationalisation of all change mechanisms specified in your theory of change.

The TiDieR-PHP reporting guideline for population health and policy interventions provides a useful framework for intervention developers to get a sense of which aspects of your intervention content should be specified (Campbell et al., 2018). This includes the rationale behind the intervention, including how intervention activities are linked to expected effects upon causal factors and outcomes, what materials are used, how the intervention was planned and delivered, who provided it, who received it, where it was provided, when and how often it was provided and aspects of its delivery, such as how well it was delivered. It should be noted that this framework is used to facilitate a transparent reporting of interventions. However, it is also a useful guide to provide intervention developers with the type of detail that is required at the stage of operationalising your theory of change. This level of detail is essential as it facilitates effective implementation and replication. If your intervention lacks detail, then it will be difficult for others to implement it. How will they know what to do or the rationale behind what they are being asked to do? If your intervention is effective, then how will others benefit from it, if they cannot apply it? It is incredibly important to be as detailed as possible.

Knowledge link: This topic is also covered in Chapter 11

Similarly to developing your theory of change, we propose that you develop your theory of action by reviewing relevant literature and drawing upon local and contextual knowledge via workshops or other, similar means. We have provided intervention development tools in previous chapters that could be drawn upon during this step.

Knowledge link: This topic is also covered in Chapters 4, 5 and 6

Decisions as to how you operationalise your theories of change should be guided by consideration of:

1. Assumptions
2. Available resources
3. Evidence of effectiveness (what has worked before and in other settings)
4. Acceptability
5. Sustainability
6. Ethical considerations and unintended consequences.

Assumptions

The development of programme theory requires that assumptions be made explicit. Your goal is to develop a theory of action that is as free of assumptions as possible. This may not always be possible. In such cases, contingency plans should be put in place to mitigate against any potential situations that should arise if your assumptions do not hold.

Consider 'availability of appropriate facilities and supplies' from Figure 7.1. This change mechanism proposes that the provision of increased handwashing facilities, soap and masks, and so on, will result in an increase in protective behaviour. There is an assumption underpinning this change mechanism that there will be enough supplies, and that people will have access to these supplies and facilities at the right time and place. However, this assumption is based on functional systems such as manufacturing, marketing and distribution. There is also an assumption that individuals will make use of the available facilities and supplies. However, can we be confident that they will do so? If you are applying this change mechanism in a culture that operates on authoritarian principles, then you might be fairly certain that people will use the facilities and supplies if they are told to do so. However, if you are applying this change mechanism in a culture that is non-authoritarian, the assumption begins to look less certain, since members of such a population may be less likely to adhere to instruction. This uncertainty represents a risk to the success of your intervention. How might you mitigate against this risk? Could you somehow incentivise the use of facilities? Or enforce their use? These are the types of practicalities that you must think about, but they may come with ethical concerns.

It is always good practice to identify and test your assumptions. The extent to which you can do this will depend on the resources available to you. However, it is usually possible for this to be done in three main ways:

1. Conducting primary research (gathering your own data)
2. Identifying relevant research literature – research which has previously tested the assumptions in question
3. Consulting and brainstorming with stakeholders

Conducting primary research (gathering your own data)

Throughout this book we have emphasised the importance of gathering your own data to inform the development of your intervention. This could take the form of interviews, focus groups, surveys, workshops, or case studies. In some cases, primary research may not be necessary since the assumption has been tested widely in the research literature. However, the context may be sufficiently different as to warrant the collection of your own data to see if the assumption holds.

Identifying relevant research literature: studies or reports that have previously tested the assumption in question

It is possible that someone may have already tested the assumption. A useful starting point is to identify any relevant literature reviews. Literature reviews are an excellent starting point since it is likely that someone else may have researched the assumption in question, saving you a lot of work in the process. As described earlier in this book, literature search tools and electronic journals are readily available if you are based in an academic institution. If you are based outside of academia, it is possible to search for broad literature overviews online. It is fairly common practice for researchers to post copies of their work online in university repositories – these are free to access and can usually be accessed by typing the name of the paper into a search engine. Alternatively, you may find useful summaries of the literature to guide your decision making on the websites of major health bodies, for example the National Health Service, the National Institute for Health and the World Health Organization.

Consulting stakeholders

Knowledge link:
This topic is
also covered in
Chapter 2

As acknowledged in previous chapters, good intervention development practice requires adequate representation of the needs and interests of stakeholders and we recommend that interventions are co-produced. The input of your team and wider stakeholders is extremely valuable at this stage as they will be able to draw upon their local knowledge and contextual experience as to whether your assumptions are likely to hold. In some respects, this is far more valuable than testing an assumption on the basis of a research paper written by someone who is not familiar with context in which your intervention will be implemented. Your team and wider stakeholders are intimately familiar with context and how any relevant systems work and interact with one another. They should be able to spot potential problems quickly and be able to advise on how to mitigate any potential negative effects if assumptions do not hold. Suggestions for how to mitigate against any potential negative effects are also likely to be highly effective since these will draw upon contextual knowledge. Similar to other sections of this book, we would advise utilising workshops to seek stakeholder feedback. We have presented a number of intervention tools throughout this book that could be used as part of such a workshop. You may also wish to consult with wider stakeholders, using interviews or focus groups. If you are pressed for resources, conversations with your team and informal conversations with wider stakeholders are an alternative method.

Knowledge link:
This topic is
also covered in
Chapters 4, 5
and 6

To illustrate the points in this section, let's take a look at another of the change mechanisms outlined in Figure 7.1: 'Individual level – Education and practical guidance (about the virus, its consequences, how it is transmitted and protective behaviours)'. This change mechanism assumes that people will behave accordingly if they have sufficient knowledge of the virus and what they must do to protect themselves. We need to identify how to test this assumption. A good starting point here is to identify whether there are any literature reviews or overviews which have tested this assumption previously. This assumption makes a general statement around human behaviour in relation to health. It supposes that knowledge of health issues and protective behaviours is sufficient to change behaviour.

Within the research literature, there are multiple studies and literature reviews of relevance (Coates et al., 2008). Since the problem we are focusing on is a virus, it would make sense to look to see if this assumption has been tested in relation to other viruses. A relatively recent comparison might be found in relation to HIV (although modes of transmission differ to that of COVID-19, a respiratory illness). Many of the early HIV prevention campaigns focused on providing members of the public with information about the virus to provoke fear, alongside a recommendation to practise safer sex using condoms. Many of these campaigns were ineffective, with those involved concluding that knowledge, whilst necessary, is not sufficiently protective in and of itself. In other words, if people are unaware that they should use a condom, then it is unlikely that they will do so. If they are aware that they should use a condom, then it is more likely that they will, but only if they are supported by other interventions. In the case of HIV, these other interventions include provision of free condoms, sexual health tests and skill building. Intervention developers also recognised that sex is a positive, enjoyable and intimate aspect of many people's identity. They therefore aimed to make condom use more attractive by linking any messaging around HIV prevention to this more positive message, compared to focusing on instilling fear.

Many studies have reported that knowledge is not sufficient to change behaviour when it comes to many health issues (Kelly and Barker, 2016). In relation to the problem of COVID-19, we can clearly see the benefit of knowledge in preventing its spread. Individuals need to know how it is transmitted, the health consequences of contracting the virus and any protective measures that they can employ. However, having looked at the research literature, we now know that this is insufficient in and of itself and that provision of knowledge must be supported by other interventions. In other words, it is not enough to tell people about the virus and what they can do to protect themselves. Looking at Figure 7.1, we can see four other change mechanisms which might support the provision of knowledge, such as providing members of the public with access to handwashing supplies. As previously stated, however, we must mitigate against any assumptions that may underpin these – for example, that people will use these supplies if they are provided with access to them.

The finding that knowledge is insufficient to change behaviour is so broad and universally accepted that stakeholder input is probably not required to test this assumption. However, change mechanisms which are highly contextual will require stakeholder input as a necessity. For example, the theory of change outlined in Figure 7.1 proposes contact tracing as a change mechanism. This refers to identifying new infections in the community and subsequently informing close contacts to stop and prevent further spread. The success of this relies on the assumption that people will isolate once they have been informed that they have the virus. However, in areas of poverty, this might mean losing access to social support and losing income. Stakeholder input is of huge value in identifying potential issues here and any solutions to such issues that may arise.

Activity 7.1

Critical thinking

For each of the change mechanisms outlined in Figure 7.1, consider what assumptions have been made and how these might affect how the intervention is implemented in practice. How might you mitigate against any negative effects should these assumptions not hold?

Available resources and assets

How you operationalise your change mechanisms will depend a great deal on the resources and assets that you have available to you. A resource (asset) is any tangible or non-tangible support that could be called upon or used in the intervention development process. It stands to reason that the more resources you have at your disposal – financial, human and community resources – the more options will be available to you regarding how you operationalise your intervention. For example, an intervention developer with limited financial resources at his or her disposal may need to think creatively about how they could draw upon goodwill and existing community resources to implement their intervention. This again emphasises the importance of stakeholders. Forming these relationships early can often give access to resources at no to little cost.

Resources can be categorised in terms of who is involved in your project and what skills or access they can offer, and what physical resources are available to you (funding, staff time, venues, etc.). Another way to conceptualise resources is to think of them as assets that will increase the likelihood of success in tackling the problem. These can be:

- economic, e.g. funding
- physical, e.g. environmental, space
- community, e.g. local groups, the existing infrastructure, community members
- human resources within a system, e.g. capacity, time, staff
- cultural, e.g. faith-based organisations, cultural values
- stakeholders.

It can be helpful to develop an asset map. These are tools for documenting the available assets that, in this case, can be drawn on to operationalise your theory of change. There are various tools for asset mapping, especially for those developing community-based interventions (e.g. Public Health Foundation, 2010). For example, it can be useful (depending on the intervention of course) to consider institutions or organisations within the community which could be helpful (e.g. libraries, churches, businesses); the skills and capacities of those in the community or those involved in delivery of the intervention;

or any physical spaces in which community members congregate or come together, since these could potentially be utilised as part of your intervention.

Activity 7.2

Reflection

How might resources affect the implementation of interventions aimed at reducing the spread of coronavirus, shown in Figure 7.1?

Evidence of effectiveness

First and foremost, for each proposed activity, you should ask yourself whether it is likely to trigger your theory of change. As you operationalise your theory of change into activities, you should seek to do so by drawing on evidence related to what has worked previously. We appreciate that, in some circumstances, there will be a need for novel intervention. In such circumstances, you should rely on the remainder of the consid-erations outlined in this section. For the most part, however, there will be at least some evidence that you can draw upon from similar work that has been conducted, whether it be published research data or data at a local level. It is incredibly useful at this stage, pos-sibly as part of workshop activities with your stakeholders, to understand what has been done previously or what currently is being done to tackle the problem in the community. This could give you an on-the-ground, real-world insight as to what has been done and how it was received. This exercise might help you to avoid repeating previous mistakes.

To illustrate how evidence of effectiveness can inform the operationalisation of change mechanisms, let's look again at our COVID-19 example: legislation; and education/practical guidance.

Legislation

By the middle of March 2020, many Asian countries as well as some European nations had begun to legislate national lockdowns to control the spread of COVID-19. These lockdowns essentially introduced curbs in relation to household mixing and legislation related to how many times and for what reason members of the public could leave their home. By mid-March 2020, there was growing evidence that national lockdowns appeared to be effective for preventing the exponential growth of the virus. This was evident in the public health reports of affected countries – if you disrupt transmission, you will prevent the spread of the virus. Within Europe, Italy was the first country to apply such a lockdown. Upon seeing the impact of national lockdowns on the spread of the virus, many countries began to adopt a similar approach, albeit tailored to specific cultural and social circumstances.

Education/practical guidance

As we stated earlier, there is evidence demonstrating that education is necessary but not sufficient to change individual behaviour. In the case of COVID-protective behaviours – such as handwashing, mask wearing and cough hygiene – education is of course important since individuals need to be aware of what they can do to protect themselves and others before these behaviours can occur. Earlier, we described how other interventions are necessary alongside education for it to have any effect. In our COVID-19 example, multiple interventions (e.g. legislation) are delivered alongside education/practical guidance. Additionally, a body of literature exists that identifies how best to deliver information and practical guidance. We know from the research literature that practical guidance must be specific and clear for it to be effective (Bonell et al., 2020). Many public health campaigns around coronavirus were therefore tailored with specific and clear messaging. For example, in the United Kingdom, the slogan 'Stay at home: protect the NHS' provided clear instruction. A later variation on this messaging – 'Stay alert, control the virus, save lives' – became far less specific and arguably less useful.

Whether an intervention has been shown to be effective or not is important information for intervention development. It is also important to identify whether there is any evidence relating to a similar group, setting or context to your own. This literature – if it exists – may contain important information, including whether any tweaks to the intervention were required to bolster effectiveness, and any unintended consequences which we will cover shortly.

Acceptability

Knowledge link: This topic is also covered in Chapter 2

Acceptability refers to the extent to which people delivering or receiving an intervention consider it to be appropriate or acceptable. If those delivering or receiving the intervention find it to be unacceptable, the chances of its successful implementation and subsequent attainment of intended outcomes are reduced. It is important to note that what is acceptable for one group, setting or context may not be acceptable in another. The acceptability of your activities can be explored as part of workshop activities with your stakeholders. Suggestions at this stage can result in tweaks that may increase acceptability, or alternative ideas as to how to operationalise your change mechanisms.

You may also need to consider acceptability to policy makers and those in power. Depending on the politics of both national and local government, it may be difficult to implement politically unpalatable interventions. Many such interventions are related to public health problems which are viewed as having a moral dimension, such as alcohol and drug misuse. Conservative governments, for example, may deliver more punitive and/or ineffective interventions (e.g. criminalising drug use) rather than interventions which may be effective yet perceived to be too 'soft', against their moral principles or too liberal. One such example would be establishing medically supervised drug consumption rooms (DCRs) in areas with high levels of injecting drug users.

Sustainability

One of the principles of intervention development is to build sustainability into your intervention. It is good practice to aim to develop an intervention that will last in the long term (Bodkin and Hakimi, 2020). Sustainability is a direct consequence of the extent to which an intervention is embedded within the systems and routines in which it operates (Proctor et al., 2011). It is essential that you incorporate consideration of sustainability both in your theory of change and as you operationalise your change mechanisms. One of the many benefits of co-producing an intervention is that activities are developed with the foresight of individuals with knowledge of the systems in which they will be implemented. Those individuals have a far greater sense of what is likely to be sustainable in that context than someone external to the system. As outlined earlier in this book, failure to create a sustainable intervention can have a negative impact on the morale of the participants involved. By working closely with your team and working with wider stakeholders to identify ways in which the intervention can coexist within existing systems and routines, your intervention has a greater chance of surviving and thriving in the long run.

Knowledge link: This topic is also covered in Chapters 2 and 6

Ethical considerations and unintended consequences

As we have emphasised, you should consider the ethical implications of any decisions you make as you develop your intervention. In relation to developing your theory of action, this should involve consideration of any specific activities that you are proposing. The issues around sustainability and assumptions covered in previous sections have ethical implications – that of damaged participant morale if sustainability is not built into intervention development and potential harms if assumptions are not properly mitigated against. You should consider each proposed activity and whether there is a potential for harm. If you identify a potential for harm, you must outline how you will mitigate against

Knowledge link: This topic is also covered in Chapters 2, 5, 6 and 7

it or operationalise your theory of change in a different way. Again, this is something that benefits greatly from co-production since those you are working with have local knowledge that can both help to identify potential issues (that you may not have otherwise spotted if working alone) and provide sustainable solutions.

Interventions to reduce the spread of COVID-19 have a number of ethical implications and unintended consequences. First, many of these interventions can be viewed as curbing our freedoms – our right to travel, to mix with others, to socialise and to work. Despite this, we have seen that such drastic interventions have the desired effect on the spread of the virus. This is evident in data presented at government briefings across the globe. It is important to consider that these interventions create unintended consequences in and of themselves. For example, placing restrictions on our social lives may cause loneliness, remove social support from those that need it most in communities, and potentially contribute to increased alcohol and substance abuse. Similarly, the mobilisation of health services towards the virus may impact on health services in relation to other conditions such as cancer and heart disease. There is therefore a balance to be maintained between intervening and managing any harms which may inadvertently come from this. It is not sufficient to simply accept the harms. It is necessary to try to mitigate against these.

Activity 7.3

Reflection

What might the unintended consequences be of the following COVID-19 interventions? How might you mitigate against these?

- closure of schools to reduce the spread of coronavirus
- closure of care homes and facilities to protect the vulnerable
- installation of alcohol hand gel and soap facilities across community settings
- asking the population to stay at home unless it is absolutely necessary to go outside
- mass media campaign to raise awareness of the severity of the virus and protective behaviours
- fast-tracked safety trials for potential vaccines.

INTERVENTION FIDELITY AND THE NEED FOR FLEXIBILITY

Much has been written in recent times about the importance of fidelity to intervention delivery (Perez et al., 2016). Much of this literature argues that the activities that make up interventions should be followed precisely as 'prescribed', in some cases necessitating vast manuals and scripts for those delivering these. Many such interventions are licensed and sold commercially, with the argument put forward that instructions must be followed to the letter in order for said interventions to be effective. The danger with this approach is that too much rigour can be harmful to the success of an intervention. The one-size-fits-all approach disregards the need for interventions to be tailored to local context. For example, many US-based parenting programmes are written with US culture in mind. Implementing these in the UK would require adaptation. Yet, many such interventions do not allow for this.

We argue that there needs to be greater flexibility when it comes to how interventions are designed and implemented. We propose that theoretical fidelity (i.e. fidelity to the theory of change) should remain the same across settings and systems. Practical fidelity (i.e. fidelity to the theory of action) is likely to differ across settings. This is because what works in one setting or system may require adaptation in another for it to be effective. Theory of change and theory of action essentially explain the same thing but at different levels of explanation. Theory of change requires identifying your change mechanisms and how you expect them to influence your outcomes. Theory of action requires identifying and planning how you will activate these change mechanisms in practice. Theory of action, by its nature, requires consideration of context.

Activity 7.4

Planning

The government has prepared guidance in relation to reducing the incidence of coronavirus infections in care homes whilst ensuring that residents have meaningful contact with friends and loved ones. The guidance was developed with input from care home providers, family and friends, public health teams and third-sector organisations. The theory of change underpinning the guidance consists of four change mechanisms:

- personal protective equipment for care home staff and visitors
- routine testing for care home staff
- testing for designated visitors
- vaccination of residents and staff.

(Continued)

The guidance recognises that, whilst the change mechanisms should remain the same (theory of change) across care homes, the way that these are operationalised (theory of action) will need to be designed at a local level by individual care homes themselves.

1. For each change mechanism, generate a list of questions to help individual care homes operationalise these into specific activities.
2. Plan a workshop that individual care homes could use to develop a theory of action. Specify:

   • who you will recommend that care homes invite to the workshop and why
   • the intervention development tools you will use, and why these are appropriate.

MAPPING YOUR THEORY OF ACTION

The previous chapter introduced logic models – these are essentially a chain of outcomes at the heart of programme theory. They display hypothesised cause-and-effect relationships between change mechanisms and short-, medium- and long-term outcomes. Once you have identified activities to trigger your outcome chains, you can add these to your logic model. Taken together, your logic model now represents your theory of change (change mechanisms and how they relate to outcomes) and your theory of action (activities to trigger change mechanisms). We will close this chapter by using the example of Stand Up For Health to illustrate this, since we have used this case study in the previous two chapters.

CASE STUDY: STAND UP FOR HEALTH

The previous chapter described the theories of change underpinning Stand Up For Health – an intervention to reduce workplace sedentary behaviour (see Figure 7.2).

The theories of change underpinning Stand Up For Health are listed at the left of the outcomes chain, shown in Figure 7.2. Note that these are listed as occurring at different levels of change, from individual behaviour change to organisational-level change. These theories of change were identified by drawing on a mix of scientific theory and working theory. For example, intervention developers propose that goal-setting and the provision of incentives (the mechanism of change) will increase motivation, which will in turn lead

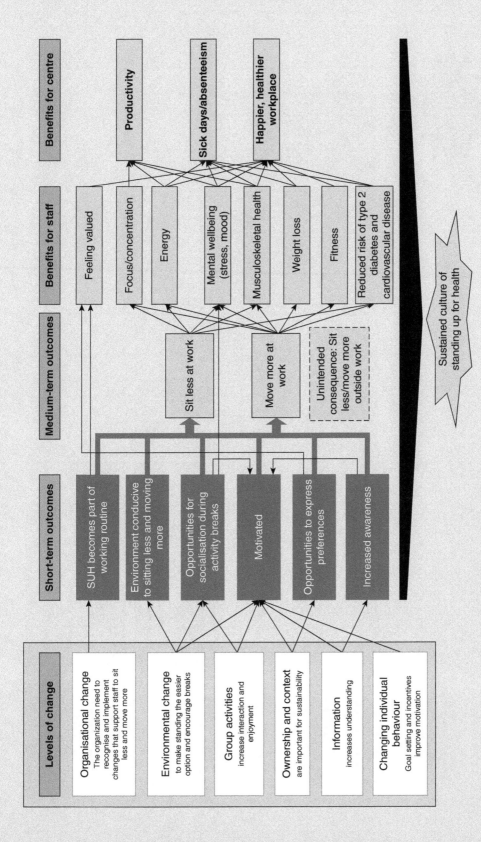

Figure 7.2 Stand Up For Health logic model including mechanisms of change

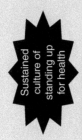

Sustained culture of standing up for health

Individual behaviour
- Motivational techniques – goal setting (weight loss, fitness, steps)
- Desk-based stretches
- Token system (where individuals get tokens for meeting targets and work towards centre goals)

Information
- Website
- Delivery of messages

Ownership and context
- Initial event prioritising outcomes
- SUH committee includes staff from all levels
- Making sure all activities are fit for purpose

Group activities
- Charity run/walks
- Walking/running groups
- Team-based activities
- Competitions
- Yoga/Tai Chi classes
- Bingo

Environmental change
- Equipment from SUH team
- Placement of equipment and designated SUH spaces
- Changes to desk structure

Key Element

Organisational change
- SUH committee
- Action plan
- Included in induction
- Changes to working routine
- Supervisor buy-in

Levels of change

Changing individual behaviour
Goal setting and incentives improve motivation

Information
increases understanding

Ownership and context
are important for sustainability

Group activities
increase interaction and enjoyment

Environmental change
to make standing the easier option and encourage breaks

Organisational change
The organisation recognises and implements changes that support staff to sit less and move more

Figure 7.3 Stand Up For Health: theory of action

to sitting less and moving more at work, which will in turn lead to a number of benefits for staff, including increased focus, concentration and fitness, in addition to wider benefits for the centre. You can see specific outcome chains by looking at the arrows. The mechanism of change in this instance is informed by goal-setting theory and operant learning theory. Similarly, intervention developers propose that recognition and implementation of changes which support staff to sit less and move more will lead to Stand Up For Health becoming part of the working routine. The intervention developers hypothesise that this will lead directly to staff feeling valued and a happier, healthier workplace in the longer term. It will also directly lead to staff sitting less and moving more at work and a number of long-term outcomes. The mechanism of change in this instance is informed by stakeholder views as to how best to trigger this outcomes chain – working theory. The theory of action (i.e. activating activities) for each theory of change is shown in Figure 7.3. These were informed both by stakeholder consultation and evidence of effectiveness.

Figure 7.3 shows the operationalisation of change mechanisms at multiple levels of intervention. For example, activities at the organisational level include the development of organisational action plans, and changes to working routine. Similarly, activities at the individual level include the introduction of desk-based stretches and the application of goal-setting. Due to space limitations in the diagram, it is not possible to show any of these activities in depth. However, for each of these activities, detailed guidance as to the specifics of operationalisation (content, format, recipient, intensity and duration) was given.

SUMMARY

This chapter has described how to develop a theory of action in order to activate your underpinning theory of change. We described how to operationalise change mechanisms into activities, drawing on existing evidence and local knowledge. We demonstrated that the way an intervention is operationalised is highly dependent on the context in which you intend to implement your intervention. It is essential to examine any assumptions made as you undertake this process and either revisit and start anew or mitigate any potential harms that may arise if these do not hold. A good theory of action should specify intervention activities in as much detail as possible, including the underpinning rationale, in order to facilitate implementation and increase the likelihood of your intervention's success. Whilst developing your theory of action, you must consider assumptions, the available resources, evidence of effectiveness, acceptability, sustainability, and any ethical considerations and unintended consequences.

FURTHER READING

Bodkin, A., and Hakimi, S. (2020) 'Sustainable by design: a systematic review of factors for health promotion program sustainability', *BMC Public Health*, 20: 964.

Campbell, M., Katikireddi, S. V., Hoffmann, T., Armstrong, R., Waters, E., and Craig, P. (2018) 'TIDieR-PHP: a reporting guideline for population health and policy interventions', *British Medical Journal*, 361.

REFERENCES

Bodkin, A., and Hakimi, S. (2020) 'Sustainable by design: a systematic review of factors for health promotion program sustainability', *BMC Public Health*, 20: 964.

Bonell, C., Michie, S., Reicher, S., West, R., Bear, L., Yardley, L., Curtis, V., Amlot, R., and Rubin, G. J. (2020) 'Harnessing behavioural science in public health campaigns to maintain "social distancing" in response to the COVID-19 pandemic: key principles', *Journal of Epidemiology and Community Health*, 74 (8): 617–19.

Campbell, M., Katikireddi, S. V., Hoffmann, T., Armstrong, R., Waters, E., and Craig, P. (2018) 'TIDieR-PHP: a reporting guideline for population health and policy interventions', *British Medical Journal*, 361.

Coates, T. J., Richter, L., and Caceres, C. (2008) 'Behavioural strategies to reduce HIV transmission: how to make them work better', *The Lancet*, 372 (9639): 669–84.

Kelly, M. P., and Barker, M. (2016) 'Why is changing health-related behaviour so difficult?', *Public Health*, 136: 109-16.

Perez, D., Van der Stuyft, P., Zabala, M. C., Castro, M., and Lefevre, P. (2016) 'A modified theoretical framework to assess implementation fidelity of adaptive public health interventions', *Implementation Science*, 11: 91.

Proctor, E., Silmere, H., Raghavan, R., Hovmand, P., Aarons, G., Bunger, A., Griffey, R., and Hensley, M. (2011) 'Outcomes for implementation research: conceptual distinctions, measurement challenges, and research agenda', *Administration and Policy in Mental Health and Mental Health Services, 38* (2): 65–76.

Public Health Foundation (2010) Healthy People Toolkit: A Field Guide to Health Planning. *Developed by the Public Health Foundation, under contract with the Office of Disease Prevention and Health Promotion, Office of Public Health and Science*. Washington, DC: US Department of Health and Human Services, p. 71.

ACTIVITY ANSWERS

Activity 7.1: Critical thinking

Population level – legislation (e.g. to introduce national or local lockdowns, limits on social freedoms)

1.   Assumption – People will follow rules despite this potentially having an impact on their income and social relationships.

2.   Mitigation – Reduce the negative impact of legislation and increase the likelihood of compliance by compensating affected workers; foster a collective sense of responsibility to look after the vulnerable and loved ones; introduce punitive measures.

Population and community level – Social norms (to establish new, accepted protective behaviours)

- Assumption – Implies that people will readily adopt protective behaviours.
- Mitigation – Foster a collective sense of responsibility to look after the vulnerable and loved ones. Emphasise the effectiveness of the protective behaviours. Provision of clear guidance.

Community level – Contact tracing (to identify new infections in the community and prevent further spread)

1.   Assumption – People will be happy to forgo their privacy in order to have their contacts and movements traced.
2.   Mitigation – Foster a collective sense of responsibility to look after the vulnerable and loved ones; introduce punitive measures.

Environmental level – The availability of appropriate facilities and supplies (e.g. hand-washing stations, disinfectant and face masks)

- Assumption – People will use facilities and supplies safely and adequately if they are provided with these.
- Mitigation – Provision of clear guidance on how to use facilities and supplies safely.

Individual level – Education and practical guidance (about the virus, its consequences, how it is transmitted and protective behaviours)

- Assumption – People will do as they have been asked.
- Mitigation – Foster a collective sense of responsibility to look after the vulnerable and loved ones. Emphasise the severity and consequences of the virus. Emphasise the effectiveness of protective behaviours. Provision of clear guidance.

Activity 7.2: Reflection

Legislation that introduces punitive measures for breaking lockdown rules (fines, etc.) will require policing and judicial resources. Provision of education and practical guidance will require considerable financial resources if using mass media communication. More tailored education and guidance may require human resources (staff and time) to develop and deliver this.

Activity 7.3: Reflection

1. Closure of schools to reduce spread of coronavirus:
   a. May impact upon learning outcomes, particularly for children from disadvantaged backgrounds/Provision of home-schooling and equipment may mitigate against this
2. Closure of care homes and facilities to protect the vulnerable during a pandemic:
   a. Increased loneliness in residents/Technology may help to mitigate against this
   b. Increased depression in residents/Engaging activities may help to mitigate against this
3. Installation of alcohol hand gel and soap facilities across community settings:
   a. Potential issues if hand gel and soap are not skin-friendly/irritants/Careful consideration of appropriate supplies needed
4. Asking the population to stay at home unless absolutely necessary to go outside:
   a. Risk of increase in unhealthy behaviours – sedentary behaviour, alcohol use, etc./ Emphasise that exercise is important and valid reason for being outdoors and ensure that health promotion services and helplines remain open
5. Mass media campaign to raise awareness of the severity of the virus and protective behaviours:
   a. Potential to cause fear in the population, particularly amongst groups most affected, which may lead to further reduced contact and reluctance to be outdoors even for essential items such as food/Careful delivery of the message required in addition to clear messaging around efficacy of protective behaviours
   b. Careful delivery of the message required in addition to clear messaging around the efficacy of protective behaviours
6. Fast-tracked safety trials for potential vaccines:
   a. May lead to concerns around vaccine safety and contribute to anti-vaxxer conspiracy theories/Consistent and clear science communication necessary

Activity 7.4: Planning

For each change mechanism, generate a list of questions to help individual care homes operationalise these into specific activities

For all change mechanisms: Care homes should consider any assumptions, sustainability of activities, in addition to ethical implications and potential unintended consequences. For example, in purchasing antibacterial hand gel, it is possible that some care homes may assume that staff and visitors will always use this. However, it is entirely possible that some staff or visitors may be allergic to some of the ingredients. Purchasing a hand gel that is less likely to irritate would solve this issue to some extent. Similarly, care homes need to think about how they can embed activities into routine practice to increase sustainability. In thinking of how to operationalise visitor testing and limits on visiting time, they need to consider the potential unintended consequences of placing limits on the time that loved ones can spend together. They therefore need to find the proper balance between restricting visiting times and resident wellbeing. Specific questions for each change mechanism include but are not limited to the following:

Personal protective equipment for care home staff and visitors, including antibacterial hand gel:

- What protective equipment is needed?
- How much is needed and how much will it cost?
- Who will supply it and how often?
- Who will monitor supplies and how often?

Routine testing for care home staff:

- What tests will be purchased and how much will they cost?
- Who will be responsible for managing and implementing the testing programme?
- What will be the procedure if a member of staff tests positive?
- Where will tests take place and on what day/time?

Testing for designated visitors, and limits on number of visitors/visitor time:

- Questions similar to routine testing for care home staff
- How long should we allow visitors to spend time with their loved one?
- Who will be responsible for the booking system?
- What will the procedure be when visitors arrive?

Vaccination of residents and staff:

- Who will be responsible for the vaccination programme?
- How will records be kept?
- What will procedures be in the event that a resident or staff member cannot be vaccinated?

Plan a workshop that individual care homes could use to develop a theory of action

Specify who you will recommend that care homes invite to the workshop and why

Care homes should seek to include wider stakeholders in the development of their theory of action. Ideally, they should establish a team consisting of key representatives of relevant parties, so that local knowledge and experience can be incorporated from the outset. In addition to this, they could develop specific activities in a workshop with a larger group of stakeholders. Possible stakeholders include residents' relatives and friends, since they will be directly affected by the intervention; representatives from the local public health team, since they have knowledge related to PPE, testing and the local picture in relation to the virus; and third-sector carer organisations since these can also represent the voice of the resident and family and friends.

Intervention development tools you will use, and why these are appropriate

Care homes could split workshop attendees into smaller groups to brainstorm answers to the specific questions above. Brainstorming is a good method for generating a list of responses for discussion. These could be written on Post-its or cards and displayed at the front of the wider group. The facilitator could group any that are similar, then the group could have a wider discussion around any assumptions that are being made, issues pertaining to unintended consequences and ethical consideration, sustainability and acceptability. As the conversation progresses, the facilitator could facilitate agreement in relation to what each change mechanism should look like in practice. By arriving at this through discussion of the issues above, specific activities should have a greater chance of being sustainable, acceptable and less likely to cause unintended consequences.

8

6SQUID STEP 5: TESTING AND ADAPTING THE INTERVENTION

Learning objectives

After reading this chapter, you will:

- Understand why testing and adaptation are an important precursor to implementation
- Understand what should be tested and how to do so.

Scenario 8.1

Coronavirus prevention intervention in a care home

Sidra is the manager of a care home for adult residents aged between 18 and 75 years old with complex health needs, such as neurological disorders. Sidra establishes a team to co-produce an intervention using the 6SQuID framework to prevent coronavirus infections in the home, something taken extremely seriously given the vulnerable nature of residents. Her team consists of a member of the local public health team, care home staff from the four units that comprise the care home (each unit varies in its focus, with two units focusing on residents with intensive treatment needs, and two focusing on residents with less

(Continued)

Knowledge link:
This topic is
also covered in
Chapter 6

Knowledge link:
This topic is
also covered in
Chapter 7

intensive treatment needs), representatives of residents' family and friends, and physicians at the local hospital who are responsible for residents' wider care needs. After following 6SQuID steps 1–4, they have operationalised four change mechanisms (theory of change) into specific activities (theory of action). A simplified version of this is shown in Table 8.1.

Table 8.1   Change mechanisms and activities for prevention of coronavirus in care homes

Change mechanisms	Activities
Raising awareness of coronavirus and protective behaviours	*For staff*: Half-day online workshops led by a senior nursing member of staff, providing guidance around coronavirus and preventive behaviours; posters and leaflets in staff areas.
	For visitors: Staff will remind visitors of the importance of PPE and handwashing.
Personal protective equipment for care home staff and visitors	Twice-monthly deliveries of PPE; two senior staff members responsible for monitoring stock levels and ordering PPE; spot checks to ensure PPE being worn.
Routine testing for care home staff	Twice-weekly lateral flow testing within 30 minutes of arrival; testing co-ordinated by a member of staff on each care unit; testing to occur in the reception area prior to staff beginning their shift.
Visitor testing, PPE and meaningful contact for designated visitors	Visitors are required to take a lateral flow test upon arrival and wait 30 minutes until their result is received before entering; visits limited to one hour and visitors are asked to wear PPE.
Vaccination of residents and staff	Vaccination to be coordinated by senior members of staff on each of the four care units, liaising closely with the local public health team.

As part of the intervention development process, the team has worked closely with wider stakeholders to consider issues such as acceptability, sustainability, the effectiveness of proposed activities, alignment of these activities within the system of the care home and potential unintended consequences. Whilst team members have considered these issues and built these considerations into their intervention, they still need to test the intervention on a small scale to see how it works in practice and make any necessary adaptations.

INTRODUCTION

Previous chapters have walked you through the process of developing a prototype of your intervention. We refer to the intervention as a prototype at this stage because it is essentially untested in complete form. Throughout steps 1–4, we have emphasised the importance of acceptability, sustainability, the effectiveness of proposed activities, alignment of these activities within the systems in which they will be implemented and potential unintended consequences. To further optimise the effectiveness of your intervention, it is essential to test your activities in practice to identify whether they work as intended and, if not, to make the necessary adaptations. It is also likely that you will have uncertainties about aspects of the intervention that can only be answered through testing how it works in practice. This step of the 6SQuID framework describes how to go about this process.

In our opening scenario, Sidra's team could test any number of elements of her intervention. For example, workshops to raise awareness of coronavirus and protective behaviours could be tested to identify how well people engage with them and how well the material presented is understood; and the delivery plan around PPE could be tested to identify whether the system Sidra's team has developed to monitor stock levels and order additional stock, works as intended. Is the intervention sustainable? Is it acceptable? Does it align with the existing care home system? Is there fidelity to the theory of change, i.e., do the activities trigger the change mechanisms specified? It is important to note that Sidra's team has worked hard through steps 1–4 to ensure that the answer to these questions is yes. However, the team still needs to ascertain to what extent this works in practice, and to make refinements, if necessary, prior to full implementation.

Testing involves piloting and feasibility. The terms 'pilot' and 'feasibility' are often used interchangeably, however their definitions and use are actually quite different. According to the UK National Institute of Health and Research (NIHR, 2019), pilot studies are 'a version of the main study that is run in miniature to test whether the components of the main study can all work together'. They focus on testing whether the processes involved, as specified in your theory of action, can all run smoothly. The UK NIHR define feasibility studies as 'pieces of research done before a main study in order to answer the question "Can this study be done?"' Feasibility studies are concerned with testing, for instance, the willingness of participants to be randomised, acceptability of the intervention to specific participants and adherence rates. Therefore, a feasibility study asks whether a study can be carried out and, if so, how it might be done. A pilot study asks the same questions, but it is more concerned about specific design issues within the *whole* study, typically taking place in a miniature form.

Testing is a repeated process and may require some iterations before your team is satisfied that the intervention is ready to be implemented in full. This continuous process of testing and refinement is sometimes referred to as formative evaluation. Take your time at this stage, if possible – proper testing will increase the likelihood that your intervention will work as intended when implemented on a larger scale. As you work through steps 1–4, questions will undoubtably arise in relation to aspects of your intervention that you may wish to gather data to answer. For example, in developing your theory of action, you may wish to do some testing of ideas around certain activities. In practice, testing can occur at any point during the intervention development process, much as you can move between steps in the framework in general. However, it is usually standard practice to have a period of testing once you have developed a full intervention prototype, which you should have by Step 4. It is also not unheard of for interventions to be tweaked as they are being implemented further down the line, since it is good practice to monitor their implementation.

Knowledge link: This topic is also covered in Chapter 9

We will now briefly touch on some of the methods you might use as part of your testing. We will then discuss what to consider when applying these methods. We will talk about how to plan a programme of testing, and how to make refinements to your intervention. The chapter will close with some consideration of testing in relation to evaluation methods.

PROCESS EVALUATION METHODS

Process evaluation is a form of evaluation that focuses upon *how* an intervention is implemented and operates (Moore et al., 2015). It is concerned with how an intervention influences change in individuals, communities and organisations. Process evaluation explores whether the mechanism of change is working as intended, how people respond to an intervention and what influence context has on the intervention. You can also begin to explore implementation at this point, and this is where fidelity to the theory of change can be examined in more detail. It's about exploring process – what goes on in the infamous 'black box' of intervention implementation, as seen in Figure 8.1.

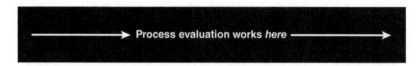

Figure 8.1   Process evaluations and the black box of intervention implementation

Process evaluation uses both quantitative and qualitative methods, including observation, interviews, focus groups, surveys, case studies and documentary analysis. Table 8.2 shows the type of process data you could obtain using each method. We recognise that not everyone will have the resources available to conduct all or even some of these methods. In this case, record keeping and listening to the experiences of those who are delivering and receiving the intervention are useful. This is the essence of process evaluation. It can be useful to follow a framework such as RE-AIM when considering what to test in relation to your intervention (Glasgow et al., 1999). RE-AIM encourages intervention developers to consider elements of your intervention that can improve its sustainability, adoption and implementation. Whilst the framework also emphasises effectiveness and efficacy, the elements relevant to this particular step are: Reach and Engagement with the target population; Adoption by staff and settings; Implementation consistency; and Maintenance over time. We will consider these elements in addition to others in the next section.

Table 8.2   Process evaluation methods and types of data collected

Method	Type of process data collected
Observation	Observer accounts of implementation and any issues
Interviews and focus groups	In-depth deliverer and recipient experiences, opinions and perspectives on the intervention; qualitative
Surveys	Deliverer and recipient opinions and perspectives on the intervention; quantitative (and qualitative to some extent if these contain open-ended and free-response questions)
Case studies	In-depth deliverer and recipient accounts of the process of taking part in activities or the intervention as a whole; this is a qualitative method
Documentary analysis	Any written materials, diaries or accounts produced as part of the intervention; qualitative or quantitative. This could be assessed for readability, clarity and so on

WHAT TO CONSIDER WHEN TESTING YOUR INTERVENTION

Typically, developers will seek to test and refine the following characteristics of their interventions. You will be familiar with these from elsewhere in the book as we encourage consideration of these from the outset and throughout. Testing is your opportunity to gain valuable information related to how your intervention works in practice. This includes:

- theory of action and its implementation, including activities, fidelity to theory of change and assumptions
- acceptability of the intervention for those delivering and receiving it
- system alignment and practicality
- reach and engagement
- unintended consequences.

Theory of action and its implementation, including activities, fidelity to theory of change and assumptions

The previous chapter described how to operationalise your theory of change into a theory of action. This involved specifying activities – including how they will be implemented – for each change mechanism in your theory of change. Much has been written about implementation and the central role it plays in determining the outcome of your intervention. The level of implementation can affect the intervention outcomes obtained (Durlak and DuPre, 2008). Effective implementation – i.e. implementation of the intervention as you intended – is more likely to lead to an optimally effective intervention since it will more closely mirror the way you conceptualised it following steps 1–4. Testing how activities work in practice can identify such issues.

In our opening scenario, Sidra's team has operationalised the change mechanism: 'Testing and meaningful contact for designated visitors'. The team has operationalised this into an activity as part of its theory of action whereby: testing is coordinated by a member of staff on each care unit (of which there are four); testing is to occur in the reception area, with visitors to wait 30 minutes for test results prior to being allowed entry; visitors are asked to wear PPE; and visits are limited to one hour. There are various points here at which implementation of this activity could deviate from what was intended. First, the testing itself – is this done correctly as to the process and the time that visitors need to wait before being allowed entry? Second, the use of PPE by those visiting – is this worn correctly, and is all necessary PPE worn at all times, i.e. mask, gloves and apron? Third, the length of visits – is the one-hour time period adhered to? These are questions that Sidra's team should consider testing. Her colleagues could do so by observing how this works in practice, although they would likely need to attempt to do this discreetly, since individuals tend to change their behaviour if they are aware they are being observed. They could telephone visitors or speak to them directly after they have visited to ask them to describe the process. They could also ask staff members who are involved in the process to share their experiences. These are fairly simple ways for team members to identify any issues around implementation of activities specified in their theory of action. If resources permit, they could look at this through qualitative interviews with visitors and staff. Activity 8.1 describes what Sidra's team did and what she found.

Activity 8.1

Reflection

To assess the implementation of activities related to the change mechanism: 'Testing and meaningful contact for designated visitors', Sidra's team decides to speak with visitors after they have undergone the testing and visiting process. She also asks a member of reception staff to observe the testing process and report back on the extent to which it appears to be consistent with the guidance provided to staff.

By talking to visitors, Sidra's team identifies an issue with the testing process itself. Proper implementation of this aspect requires staff to prepare the test sample with activating solution. This is a process which ensures that the result will be a reliable indicator of coronavirus status, i.e. whether a visitor is positive or negative. Visitors should only be involved in swabbing their throat and nose. The swab is then passed to staff who then process the result. Poor application of this process can lead to a false negative result, i.e. someone testing negative when they are actually positive. What they discover is that staff are handing visitors the lateral flow device and asking them to prepare the solution, swab their throat and nose and process the result. In his observations of the process, the receptionist has also noticed incorrect usage of the tests and visitors' confusion around the process. This has the potential to jeopardise the intended outcome of reduced incidence of coronavirus, as poor testing could result in an outbreak if a visitor is allowed to enter the premises with a false negative result.

How might Sidra's team refine the intervention to address these issues?

Monitoring the implementation of activities can also indicate instances in which there is poor theoretical fidelity. Theoretical fidelity is about adherence to the 'essence' of the intervention, or, for the 6SQuID framework, adherence to the theory of change. Theoretical fidelity proposes that interventions should be adapted to align with the system and account for differences in context, but should not lose the active or essential components of its underpinning theory of change. An activity that has poor theoretical fidelity is one that cannot trigger the change mechanism for which it was developed. In the case of Sidra's team, she is likely to have various reports from relatives about the one-hour duration of resident visits once they begin to test this aspect of their intervention. The change mechanism underpinning this activity is: 'Testing and meaningful contact for designated visitors'. The one-hour duration may be insufficient for facilitating 'meaningful contact'. Limiting the duration of contact is potentially the opposite of what is required for meaningful contact. In that sense, we could argue that the team's activity here lacks theoretical fidelity, i.e. it is unlikely to trigger the change mechanism. The intervention could possibly be refined by the team establishing what meaningful contact means for each resident and their family and friends. This personalised approach would possibly be more likely to trigger the change mechanism, and therefore to retain theoretical fidelity.

We would encourage you to test out your activities and refine them. Often in the process of intervention development, questions will come to mind about assumptions you have made and different ways of operationalising your change mechanisms. Test these out. Refine your intervention. Test again if necessary. We have used the example of a sedentary behaviour intervention in contact centres in this book. Amongst other things, testing of activities in this case involved trying out different types of fitness equipment to find what worked best for each location where the intervention was implemented.

The previous chapter described the process of operationalising theory of change into a theory of action. As part of this process, we advised that you should identify and test any assumptions in regard to both change mechanisms and the activities you develop

Knowledge link: This topic is also covered in Chapters 5, 6, 7 and 10

Knowledge link: This topic is also covered in Chapter 7

to trigger these. We advised that the development of programme theory requires that assumptions be made explicit. Additionally, contingency plans should be put in place to mitigate against any potential situations that may arise if your assumptions do not hold. We proposed that assumptions could be tested by examining the research literature alongside working closely with your team (which should consist of those with local knowledge and experience) and wider stakeholders, in addition to implementing these in practice to see whether they hold.

Acceptability of the intervention for those delivering and receiving it

Knowledge link: This topic is also covered in Chapters 5, 6 and 7

The issue of acceptability of the intervention has been raised previously. It is essential you test the acceptability of the various components. Acceptability should be seen through the lens of those delivering and receiving the intervention. In other words: To what extent do they see the intervention as appropriate based on their experiences of delivering or receiving the intervention? In the previous section, we described a situation in which Sidra (from our opening scenario) receives communications from residents' relatives and friends about the limitations of one-hour visits. This is the type of acceptability issue that might arise in response to implementing the intervention. You would of course hope to anticipate this type of issue beforehand. However, even with all the work involved from steps 1–4, issues can emerge once you begin to observe how the intervention is received in practice. This issue around acceptability would also hopefully flag to Sidra's team that there is a lack of theoretical fidelity in this activity. Another example is in relation to the change mechanism: 'Personal protective equipment for care home staff and visitors'. Sidra's team has operationalised this with a focus on both monitoring and ordering PPE stock when needed. However, in practice team members may find that there are issues with the particular stock they are using. For example, perhaps the brand they are using is not suitable for sensitive skin. Issues like these are likely to arise when testing acceptability in practice.

Acceptability can be measured in a number of different ways, primarily focused upon data collection from those delivering or receiving the intervention. This can be informal or via more formal means if resources permit, such as interviews, focus groups or workshops.

System alignment and practicality

By following steps 1–4 correctly, you can be fairly confident that your intervention should operate within the systems in which it is implemented. First, you have co-produced your intervention and worked with wider stakeholders including those who have contextual knowledge of these systems. Second, you have developed activities in close conjunction with these stakeholders with a view to ensuring that these are aligned to contextual aspects of the systems involved. In our opening scenario, there are four different units in the care home, each of which looks after patients with varying levels of treatment needs. Two of the units focus on high-intensity care, whereas the other two units are for those residents with less-intensive care needs. Sidra's team has developed the intervention with existing care home routines in mind. However, despite being fairly confident that the intervention will operate as intended within the care home system, the team must still implement it to see how it works in practice. It may be that aspects of the intervention need to be tweaked. For example, workshops may need to be scheduled at different times; those responsible for testing may need to have additional time allocated to their schedules in order for their workload to be manageable; and they may need to refine the system for managing PPE stock levels to be more consistent with routines and schedules for managing other clinical care home stock. They also need to be careful that their activities are consistent with current government and healthcare guidance around PPE and infection prevention, so that they do not fail to adhere to these.

Activity 8.2

Reflection

The care home has four units, each with residents requiring different levels of care of varying intensity. In relation to the change mechanism: 'Testing, PPE and meaningful contact for designated visitors', the team has developed activities including the use of PPE by visitors at all times. In order to test this component of the intervention, the team speaks with visitors and staff to explore their experiences, and learns that, on high-intensity treatment units, the use of PPE is causing problems. This is because many of the residents on these units are receiving end-of-life care. Visitors are therefore removing PPE in order to spend what they consider to be meaningful time with their loved ones. This finding indicates that the intervention is not completely aligned with the care home system, since these high-intensity units differ considerably from the less-intensive units.

How might Sidra's team refine the intervention so that it aligns better with the context of the high-intensity units?

Reach and engagement

In developing your intervention, you will of course have had a target population in mind. Reach can be defined as the extent to which members of the target population engage with your intervention. As mentioned above, RE-AIM is a framework for evaluating the impact of interventions (Glasgow et al., 1999). The framework emphasises reach as an important issue to consider when testing, referring to 'the absolute number, proportion, and representativeness of individuals who are willing to participate in a given initiative, intervention, or programme and reasons why or why not'. Questions to ask at this stage include:

- Who is participating? Is the target population engaging with the intervention? Are there certain groups with in the target population that are participating more than others?
- If there are issues with participation, why? Is this due to methods for advertising and promoting the intervention? Is it due to the acceptability or accessibility of activities?

In our opening scenario, reach is likely not going to be a major issue, since all staff and individuals entering the care home will be required to take part in the intervention. However, take the example of an optional intervention to support parents to develop parenting skills. Some of the change mechanisms in such an intervention might be around skill building and social support. An intervention developer might operationalise these change mechanisms into activities such as skill-building workshops for parents in addition to regular parent support meetings held in the local community. It is beneficial for the developers to learn information about the reach of their intervention since this can be used to further optimise it. As part of testing such an intervention, developers should identify how many parents engage, who is engaging, who is not engaging and why this is or is not the case. They could achieve this by collecting data on numbers attending sessions, in addition to socio-demographic information about these individuals. They might find that those parents who attend are those who live in fairly affluent areas. In this case, there is therefore a risk of the intervention contributing to widening health inequalities. Refinements could be considered to increase the likelihood of parents from less affluent areas participating in the intervention – for instance, provision of a creche for childcare, free or discounted transport, or moving the sessions closer to places that are within walking distance of less well-off areas.

Unintended consequences

Knowledge link: This topic is also covered in Chapters 2, 5, 6 and 7

Much has been written already in the book about the importance of ethical considerations and unintended consequences. Testing provides you with an opportunity to identify unforeseen issues and to make refinements prior to full implementation. These can be identified by speaking with those who are delivering and receiving the intervention, either informally or via interviews and focus groups. In our opening scenario, a number of unintended consequences might be uncovered during implementation. For example, the vaccination of residents and staff may create a false sense of security and increase the chance that use of PPE and protective behaviours may be less well adhered to. However, some residents will not be able to receive the vaccine due to advanced health conditions or advanced age. Refinements could include updating any training to cover this important information and raising awareness of this via posters and so on, through the care home. Additionally, restrictions on visiting times and use of full PPE may affect the wellbeing of both residents and their loved ones, since both of these activities place restrictions on the quality of human interaction. Refinements could be made to the process of visiting, by ensuring that this is done on an individual basis to take account of each resident's needs.

PLANNING HOW TO TEST YOUR INTERVENTION

The levels at which the intervention will be implemented (e.g. individual, community, national) can often determine the kind of testing that would be needed. This means there could be considerable variation and degree of difficulty in testing depending on the type of intervention. Often individual- or community-level interventions may require repeated testing and adaptation. For national-level interventions, it might be difficult to undertake repeated testing and adaptation. For example, if a national-level intervention has a legislative component, you may need to consider phased, area-by-area implementation to test whilst making incremental adjustments. For instance, a national smoking ban in enclosed public places would likely require a period of incremental implementation to make any necessary refinements as part of this step. This would need to be carefully thought through since there are ethical concerns involved here. You might select one area potentially to receive the smoking ban initially, but you would have to think carefully about how to make this decision. Residents in the area may feel targeted unjustly, for example, if the area selected for this initial testing has inhabitants which are mainly of a particular income bracket, ethnicity or socio-economic group. That being said, if you've fully explored acceptability and co-produced your intervention, issues such as these should have been identified in addition to solutions.

Another issue for consideration is that of the available resources. We have talked about the importance of being aware of your available resources and the benefit of making these explicit by using methods such as asset mapping. As in the other four steps of the 6SQuID process, testing involves working closely with your team to draw on members' local knowledge and experience of how this could be done efficiently. Your testing plan should be co-produced. Members of your team will bring questions to the testing process that reflect the systems within which the intervention will be implemented. This will therefore result in the necessary questions being asked that are required to finely tune your intervention such that it is sustainable, acceptable and effective. For example, in our opening scenario, Sidra's team includes a local public health advisor. This person will bring knowledge of wider health rules and regulations – such as guidance around infection prevention in health and social care settings – which they can use to generate

Knowledge link: This topic is also covered in Chapter 7

questions for testing at this stage – for example, to what extent is implementation of activities consistent with this guidance?

If you are implementing your intervention in different contexts, you should treat each of these contexts separately as part of your testing. As we have described, specific activities are likely to vary across contexts. What is important is that they should retain fidelity to the theory of change. If you are working with different contexts, it makes sense to separate testing for each of these, since your findings in one context may not be applicable to another. This can even apply to different contexts within the same system. In our opening scenario, Sidra's care home consists of four wards across two very different contexts – one with residents who have high-intensity treatment needs and another with lower-intensity needs. Her team needs to consider this when testing.

Activity 8.3

Active transport intervention

Oliver works for a local active transport charity and has developed an intervention to increase cycling and other forms of active transport in a local area with high car usage. After following steps 1–4 of 6SQuID, he has operationalised his change mechanisms into specific activities, as shown in Table 8.3.

Table 8.3   Change mechanisms and activities

Change mechanism	Activities
Improvements in cycling infrastructure – both personal and community-level	The charity will hold monthly free bicycle-repair workshops at a local park where community members can bring their bikes for a tune-up; main roads will have painted cycle lanes added.
Awareness-raising and confidence-building about cycling	A promotional campaign will take place over social media to educate drivers about safe-driving practices around cyclists; people interested in cycling can sign up to a free one-hour 'cycling in the city' course to build confidence on the road.
Signage and zebra crossings/crosswalks	Additional zebra crossings will be added to the local area to promote safe walking; additional signage demonstrating popular walk and cycle loops and paths will be added.

Oliver wants to test and refine this programme in a few blocks of the city before rolling it out more widely for a more detailed evaluation.

Develop a programme of testing for the active transport intervention described in Table 8.3. What key questions would you want answered? How would you collect data? What types of data would you collect?

MAKING ADAPTATIONS TO YOUR ACTIVITIES

The findings of any testing that you conduct should be discussed with your team and, if necessary, with wider stakeholders. Adaptation is essentially a process related to content and, as we have seen throughout the book, content should be developed alongside those with local knowledge and experience. Adaptation is done by looking at the data you have gathered from testing and making agreed refinements to components of your intervention based on those data. As we have stated, testing can often occur during steps 3–4. It is standard practice to test parts of your thinking and specific activities as you move along the framework. You could go back and forward many times before you are satisfied that the intervention is optimal. In many cases, the findings of such testing will be discussed with your team members and adaptations agreed by consensus. Once you test your intervention in full, you may produce a substantial amount of data that requires consideration of multiple adaptations. In these cases, we would suggest that a workshop with wider stakeholders (if this is practical, given resources) would likely be more appropriate. This could involve presentation of the findings from your testing, discussion of areas for adaptation and possible solutions, followed by a consensus activity to agree what form any adaptations should take. This approach to content adaptation is consistent with our approach to developing content more generally across the framework in that it should be co-produced, draw upon local knowledge and experience and, in doing so, be more likely to work as intended.

TESTING ELEMENTS OF A FUTURE EVALUATION

Testing can also include a focus on aspects of a future planned evaluation. This can include consideration of issues such as recruitment, methods and materials.

Recruitment

When testing elements of your evaluation, recruitment of your target population is an important point to consider. You will need to decide whether it is more appropriate to use a convenient sample who may not be wholly representative of your target population or a sample of the target population likely to receive the intervention when it is scaled up. The choice between a convenient sample and one that is wholly representative of your target population is often dependent on the available resources. Convenience is always faster and more cost-effective. We would suggest that, in the event of limited resources, convenience sampling is fine. In terms of testing with this sample, you may want to know whether the intended population could be recruited and enrolled in the programme. An example would be if a physical activity intervention is being designed to reduce sedentary behaviour amongst young adults. You may want to test how recruitment of those who met the eligibility criteria could be maximised and whether the recruitment approach is acceptable to them. Testing your recruitment approach at this stage is important as it may highlight any potential challenges that a future outcomes evaluation may encounter, enabling you to identify strategies to overcome such challenges.

Knowledge link: This topic is also covered in Chapter 9

Interviews and focus groups

You should also consider testing any tools you have identified for data collection, since these will be central to your outcomes evaluation. Some of the possible methods you could use to collect data have already been highlighted above. However, the actual tools that may be employed by these methods may require testing. For example, you may decide to test aspects of your qualitative methods, such as your interview or focus group guides. Testing these tools would give you an opportunity to adapt and improve them. You can test these tools with those delivering and receiving the intervention. For example, in the scenario above it was suggested that, if Sidra and her team would like to find out how the change mechanism of 'Testing and meaningful contact for designated visitors' were operationalised, they may decide to speak to visitors after they have visited the care home and care home staff to understand their perspectives on the process. Various different aspects of your topic guides should be tested. For example, the testing process can help to identify whether the questions are well formulated and do not create any ambiguity amongst your respondents. Testing can be also be used to check the flow of the questions and determine whether any rearrangement may be required.

Aside from testing the tools to be used for collecting data, you may also decide to test the data collection format. This is particularly relevant when dealing with sensitive topics. For example, if you are designing an intervention to reduce alcohol consumption amongst pregnant women, it would be sensible to test whether the interview guide is more appropriate for use in one to one interviews or focus groups. Pregnant women may not feel comfortable talking about their alcohol consumption as part of a wider group.

For focus groups, you can also observe the group dynamics of how participants respond to the questions, and gauge whether adaptation will be needed with some of the questions, or you may decide that for the main evaluation one-to-one interviews are the best approach.

Questionnaires

Quantitative methods such as questionnaires should also be tested. For example, in our opening scenario, Sidra might use a survey to understand the experiences of visitors to the care home. In doing this you could either design your own questionnaire or use a pre-existing or validated questionnaire. There are many questionnaires covering numerous topics. For example, the Survey Question Bank, which is hosted at the University of Surrey and coordinated by the UK Data Archive, provides access to an online resource that gives access to a repository of questionnaires in key topic areas. Pre-existing questionnaires often provide users with information on how to interpret the findings. In terms of using a pre-existing questionnaire, let's take the example of an intervention to support parents to develop parenting skills. Since skill building is part of the intervention, you may be planning to use a pre-existing parenting skills assessment questionnaire in the main evaluation, so the testing stage would be an opportunity to test and adapt this tool, if necessary.

Knowledge link: This topic is also covered in Chapter 9

The advantage of using pre-existing questionnaires is that often a great deal of care and expertise goes into their development to ensure that they are measuring what they are meant to measure. They can save time and money since you are not designing the tool from scratch. However, care must be taken when using these. Often, these tools are designed to be used with a particular population and small changes may affect their validity. Any changes – translating a questionnaire into a different language or to slightly adapting the wording to suit the population you are using the tool with – should be done carefully. Once these changes are made, testing can help you to validate and adapt the tool accordingly.

Sometimes there may be no suitable pre-existing questionnaires for use or you may feel that a simpler more bespoke questionnaire is more appropriate. In this case, you may decide to design your own questionnaire, or possibly borrow some of the questions from pre-existing questionnaires for your own use. Designing your own questionnaire may give you more flexibility in data collection around the areas you are focusing on.

SUMMARY

This chapter has outlined the process of testing and adapting your intervention. We have emphasised the iterative nature of this process and made the point that the scale of testing often varies, from testing specific activities through to testing the full intervention as it is implemented in practice. Testing also offers you the opportunity to test some of the tools you are planning to use in the evaluation. What is tested and how it is tested will vary depending on the content and context in which your intervention is implemented. It is important that you share your findings in relation to what has and hasn't worked as this is learning which others might find useful if they are in a similar field or developing a similar intervention.

FURTHER READING

Moore, G. F., Audrey, S., Barker, M., Bond, L., Bonell, C., Hardeman, W., Moore, L., O'Cathain, A., Tinati, T., Wight, D., and Baird, J. (2015) 'Process evaluation of complex interventions: Medical Research Council guidance', *British Medical Journal*, 350.

REFERENCES

Durlak, J. A., and DuPre, E. P. (2008) 'Implementation matters: a review of research on the influence of implementation on program outcomes and the factors affecting implementation', *American Journal of Community Psychology*, 41 (3–4): 327–50.

Glasgow, R. E., Vogt, T. M., and Boles, S. M. (1999) 'Evaluating the public health impact of health promotion interventions: the RE-AIM framework', *American Journal of Public Health*, 89 (9): 1322–7.

Moore, G. F., Audrey, S., Barker, M., Bond, L., Bonell, C., Hardeman, W., Moore, L., O'Cathain, A., Tinati, T., Wight, D., and Baird, J. (2015) 'Process evaluation of complex interventions: Medical Research Council guidance', *British Medical Journal*, 350.

National Institute of Health Research (NIHR) (2019) Available at: www.nihr.ac.uk/documents/ additional-guidance-for-applicants-including-a-clinical-trial-pilot-study-or-feasibility-as-part-of-a-personal-award-application/11702 (accessed 30 September 2021).

ACTIVITY ANSWERS

Activity 8.1: Reflection

Sidra's team might refine the intervention to address these issues by: providing further training; posting clear and specific instructions regarding the testing process in the reception area (perhaps by attaching laminated posters to the walls etc.); and regular monitoring to ensure that this is being done correctly.

Activity 8.2: Reflection

Sidra's team could look to see if there is any guidance related to the implementation of coronavirus guidance and end-of-life care. She and her colleagues could then make refinements to the intervention on units where this is applicable. They could also make this process more personalised by developing a plan for each resident based on their needs, involving the resident, family and friends.

Activity 8.3: Active transport intervention

Possible key questions:

- How many people attend the cycle repair workshops and course?
- Are more people using the cycle lanes, zebra crossing and following the signage?
- Do people feel more confident cycling after attending the course?
- Do people feel safer cycling and walking around the city?

Data collection ideas:

- Lots of qualitative data would be useful for this stage of the development and testing. You could ask people for feedback after attending the cycle repair workshops and the city cycling course for refinements to the content, timings and delivery methods (e.g. online versus in-person courses).
- Another option is the use of questionnaires, but this wouldn't provide as much opportunity for suggested improvements unless free-response questions are available.
- Observation of cycling infrastructure at various points of implementation would allow you to see if people are using it appropriately or more often.

9

6SQuID STEP 6: COLLECTING SUFFICIENT EVIDENCE OF EFFECTIVENESS TO PROCEED TO A RIGOROUS EVALUATION

Learning objectives

After reading this chapter, you will be able to:

- Develop an evaluation plan for an intervention using tools like evaluability assessment
- Consider the strengths, limitations and challenges of the various methods used for evaluation
- Ensure that the evaluation approach you take is ethical, reliable and valid.

Scenario 9.1

Speed limits

Stephanie is a councillor for the City of Edinburgh and two years ago she was elected on her promise to reduce the speed limit to 20mph on most of the city's roads. The speed limits were changed to 20mph last year. The next election is on the horizon and the City Council has received lots of complaints about the 20mph scheme, so Stephanie knows that, unless she can prove that the 20mph limit has had positive impact, she won't get re-elected.

a. What does Stephanie need to know in order to prove the impact of the 20mph limit?
b. How can she ensure that any impacts identified are due to the 20mph limit and not anything else?
c. She believes that it is important to tell people the truth, so what does she need to consider when evaluating the 20mph limit and reporting the findings to make sure she has not lied to the people and wasted taxpayers' money?

INTRODUCTION

Once an intervention has been piloted, revised and is considered 'good enough' for full implementation, the final step in intervention development is to establish sufficient evidence of effectiveness to warrant wider implementation of the intervention. This could mean moving to a large-scale rigorous evaluation (which could be a randomised controlled trial, realist evaluation, stepped-wedge or natural experimental approach); or, if resources and time are constrained, as in many not-for-profit organisations (e.g. charities and the third sector), undertaking less formal evaluation as part of the move towards wider implementation. This chapter will describe how to evaluate an intervention to assess its effectiveness in a time- and cost-efficient manner, with an emphasis on the economics of scaling up an intervention.

But first, what do we mean by evaluation? Below is the definition of evaluation developed by the United Nations Evaluation Group (UNEG), which is also used by the World Health Organization:

> An evaluation is an assessment, as systematic and impartial as possible of an activity, project, programme, strategy, policy, theme, sector, operational area or institutional performance. It focuses on expected and achieved accomplishments examining the results chain, processes, contextual factors and causality, in order to understand achievements or the lack thereof. It aims at determining the relevance, impact, effectiveness, efficiency and sustainability of the interventions and contributions of the organizations of the UN system. (www.who.int/about/what-we-do/evaluation; http://uneval.org)

While this is a long and jargon-filled definition, it contains several important details about evaluation which we will explore in this chapter. First, it is notable that organisations like the United Nations and the World Health Organization have a definition of evaluation, which reflects the fact that evaluation is not specific to any one area of research or practice, and that a wide variety of activities can be evaluated (an activity, project, programme, strategy, policy, theme, sector, operational area or institutional performance). We hope to demonstrate that valuable evaluations can be taken at every scale from the local to the international. The second and third sections of this chapter will focus on how to ensure that an evaluation is 'as systematic and impartial as possible'. But prior to that you need to know what you are evaluating.

Knowledge link:
This topic is
also covered in
Chapter 8

The definition talks about *'expected and achieved accomplishments'*, meaning that you should be evaluating whether your intervention met the original objectives, whether this means evaluating outputs, outcomes or process. In the first section of this chapter, we will discuss how both the earlier steps of 6SQuID and processes like **evaluability assessment** are essential in planning an evaluation. The mention in the definition of *'achievements or the lack thereof'* and references to *relevance, impact, effectiveness, efficiency and sustainability* in the final sentence highlight that evaluation is not simply about establishing whether an intervention 'works'. It is also about other aspects of effectiveness such as sustainability – see Chapter 2 for further discussion of issues around effectiveness, and 6SQuID is designed to enable you to build relevance and sustainability into your intervention.

There are a multitude of textbooks and courses devoted to evaluation, and consequently our ambition in this chapter is to give you the important questions to ask and to introduce some important concepts related to evaluation in order that you know where to start when planning an evaluation. Before you even start to plan an evaluation, there are two questions to consider: *Why do you want to conduct an evaluation? Who is the evaluation for?* These questions are linked, as the reason you are conducting an evaluation might be that your funders or managers or stakeholders want one. Equally, you might want to conduct an evaluation for your own or your organisation's learning, to help you understand whether all your efforts have been worthwhile. These questions are important because they help to determine the scope of the evaluation. Funders might want to learn from the evaluation whether their money was wisely spent, so want an evaluation focused on economic outcomes; whereas your organisation might want to learn more about how the intervention worked and whether anyone had missed out on receiving the intervention, suggesting that the evaluation should be more focused on processes. Often, the ultimate goal of evaluation is about using the findings to improve the intervention or programme.

Activity 9.1

Why, and for whom, does Stephanie want to evaluate the 20mph limits?

Take some time to write down in a list all the reasons you can think of for why Stephanie would want to evaluate the Edinburgh 20mph limits? In a second list, write down all the people who might be the intended audience for the evaluation. Finally, draw lines between the lists to link the reasons for the evaluation with the potential audiences, considering how these might change the scope of the evaluation.

WHAT DO YOU NEED TO KNOW TO PLAN AN EVALUATION?

Now that you have a clear sense of why you want to conduct an evaluation and who the evaluation is for, there are a number of further questions you need to consider. These questions are framed in terms of the six common types of question: *What, Who, When, Where, Why* and *How* (The 5 Ws and a H). We have already asked *Why do you want to conduct an evaluation?* and in the next section of this chapter we will discuss *How to conduct an evaluation*, so that leaves *What, Who, When* and *Where to evaluate*? Each of these questions defines the scope of the evaluation, which has been determined by your previous answers on who the evaluation is for and why an evaluation is being conducted. This information is essential not just for planning the intervention, but also to budget for the evaluation.

WHAT TO EVALUATE?

This question is asking 'what is it that your intervention is meant to have changed' and what do you want to measure? The UNEG definition mentions *'results chain' and 'processes'*, highlighting that an evaluation can focus on any of the processes, outputs or outcomes of an intervention. This is where your programme theory or logic model is really important, as it should provide details of the processes, outputs and outcomes of your intervention. The reference in the UNEG definition to *'expected and achieved accomplishments'* demonstrates that you should only be attempting to evaluate the changes you intended to make (i.e. those which are in your theory of change or theory of action). The intended audience for the evaluation will help you determine what to evaluate. For example, if you want your evaluation to be adopted by a health service, you probably want to focus on health and economic outcomes; whereas the evaluation of a workplace intervention might want to focus on productivity as well as health outcomes to convince the managers to adopt the intervention more widely. It is possible to evaluate processes, outputs and outcomes in either or both quantitative (countable or measurable data) and qualitative (non-numerical data) ways. The choice to focus on quantitative or qualitative measures will determine the methods you can use in your evaluation (see later section).

Knowledge link: This topic is also covered in Chapter 8

It is important to consider evaluating the potential harms (usually unintended) caused by your intervention as well as the potential benefits. In evaluations of new medicines, these tend to be side-effects, but it can also be important to consider harms like what other opportunities (e.g. participating in an established intervention programme) participants in your intervention might be missing out on, or how else they might be using their time (e.g. losing out on income by having to take time off work to attend a smoking intervention). Consideration of harms, as well as benefits, links to economic evaluation – as mentioned above, often evaluations need to answer the question of whether the intervention was worth what it cost (sometimes called the seventh type of question *How much?*). In health we talk about this as **cost-effectiveness**, and most new healthcare interventions need to demonstrate that they are cost-effective in order to be provided to the public. This is particularly important in countries with a national or socialised health service, many of which have an organisation which determines what is cost-effective. In England, this organisation is the National Institute for Health and Care Excellence (NICE), and it has determined that interventions that cost up to £20,000 per Quality Adjusted Life Year (QALY) will be funded by the National Health Service, with different decisions determining whether more expensive interventions should be funded. If you want to undertake an economic evaluation and don't have the appropriate experience, we recommend seeking expert advice. Most textbooks on economic evaluation are focused on healthcare interventions, like Drummond et al. (2015), but will still introduce the reader to the important concepts. Any economic evaluation will compare the costs of the intervention against the benefits. So, you would need to plan how to collect these data for your intervention. At this point, and throughout this chapter, you will see that, even though this is the sixth step in 6SQuID, it can be incredibly helpful to start planning your evaluation as you are developing the intervention. You do not want to miss an opportunity to collect data such as the costs of the intervention.

Who are the participants in the evaluation?

The answer to this question will be determined by what you are going to evaluate. Ideally you want to be collecting data directly from the people experiencing the intervention and the potential benefits. But if you are conducting more of a process evaluation, you might focus more on the people delivering the intervention. Sometimes, it is either not feasible or not ethical to collect data from the intervention participants directly; for example, when they are young children or babies or those with certain health conditions (e.g. dementia without the ability to consent). Depending on the scope of your intervention, you might also be collecting data from a broader range of people and organisations. An important consideration at this point is about how much of a burden on the participants the data collection might be. For example, taking a blood sample or measuring blood pressure might not take much time, but can cause harm; completing a short survey might not take much time but you need to think about the literacy of the participants; and an interview or focus group might take a significant period of time. We will return to this in later sections.

When to evaluate it?

Knowledge link: This topic is also covered in Chapters 6 and 7

Your programme theory or logic model will help you answer this question. It might sound obvious, but you want to be conducting your evaluation as or after the process, output or outcome are likely to have happened. For example, if you wanted to measure the number of people signing on to your weight loss programme, you could be measuring that straight away, but if you wanted to measure the amount of weight participants lost you might need to wait months or years to assess whether your intervention brought about any sustainable changes in weight. You might be in a situation where your timescales are limited by whoever has asked for the evaluation, in which case your programme theory or logic model will tell you what the shorter-term outcomes, outputs or processes are on which your evaluation could focus. You might need to trade off what you evaluate against when you need to conduct the evaluation.

WHERE SHOULD THE EVALUATION BE CONDUCTED?

The setting for your evaluation might seem obvious if your intervention is taking place in a specific location, but in order to be systematic and impartial you need to ensure that the evaluation does not take place in a situation which biases the responses the participants might give. The location of the evaluation will also determine some of the costs of the evaluation and matters that you might need to consider, such as the policies and risk assessments regarding the location, which might determine how your evaluation proceeds.

Evaluability assessment

As well as defining the scope of your evaluation, these questions help you understand what evaluation is feasible. However, there is a broader range of questions to determine whether an evaluation is feasible, and these have been wrapped up together in a process called evaluability assessment. The process was proposed by Wholey in 1979 and has more recently been described by Leviton et al. (2010: 214) as 'a pre-evaluation activity designed to maximize the chances that any subsequent evaluation of programs, practices, or policies will result in useful information'. The review by Leviton et al. (2010) is an excellent source of information on evaluability assessment. Wholey (1979) originally defined six steps to an evaluability assessment:

- involving the intended users of evaluation information
- clarifying the intended program
- exploring program reality
- reaching agreement on the needed changes in activities or goals
- exploring alternative evaluation designs
- agreeing on the evaluation priorities and intended uses of information. (Leviton et al., 2010: 217)

You can see that the questions we have asked so far in this chapter and the previous steps of 6SQuID have provided information that is useful to this process. However, the experience of Leviton et al. (2010) was that Wholey (1979) made the process appear overly linear, moving through the steps in order, whereas their experience was that the process tended to become cyclical and iterative, and therefore they proposed the adapted process described in the evaluability assessment concept summary box. The approach that the authors of this book have taken to handling this cyclical and iterative process is to conduct the evaluability assessment through one or more workshops with the relevant stakeholders. You can save a lot of time by bringing everyone into the same room. The evaluability assessment process is meant to be undertaken in a relatively short time period. One by Belford et al. (2017) was undertaken as part of a Master's dissertation. Further examples of evaluability assessments can be found in the Further reading section at the end of the chapter.

Concept summary

Evaluability assessment (Leviton et al., 2010)

Working with the end users of the evaluation, work through the following processes:

1. Determine the scope of the evaluation by reviewing procedural documents and other material describing the intervention, and consulting stakeholders. Having gathered this information, if there is agreement about the goals of the intervention and evaluation, proceed to the next stage. If there is a disagreement, feed back to the intervention lead, and resolve before the evaluation and evaluability assessment can proceed.
2. Derive and agree the logic model for the intervention. During this step, you need to learn both about how the intervention is intended to work and how it is working in practice, so it is important to consult with those delivering and receiving the intervention. Any disagreement about the logic model needs to be resolved for the evaluability assessment and evaluation to proceed.
3. Write up a report explaining the assessment of the following aspects of an evaluation of the intervention:
   a. Plausibility
   b. Areas for intervention development
   c. Evaluation feasibility
   d. Options for further evaluation
   e. Critique of the quality and availability of relevant data

This information may be used to revise the intervention logic model before proceeding with any evaluation.

There are three feedback loops described in the concept summary box, two of which relate to securing agreement on the goals of the evaluation and the programme theory or logic model. If it is not possible to agree on these two points, Leviton et al. (2010) assert that it is not yet appropriate for an evaluation to go ahead. If you cannot agree what to measure or how the intervention is working then an evaluation is going to be very difficult, and further development of the intervention is needed. The final feedback loop is between the findings of the evaluability assessment and the programme theory or logic model, demonstrating how much the evaluation and the programme theory are linked.

The outcomes of an evaluability assessment are shown in the final process in the concept summary box. The information about the plausibility and feasibility of an evaluation and the various options which could be used to evaluate the intervention are really helpful in deciding how to proceed. However, you can also see that an evaluability assessment alone can provide useful information for programme development, and the authors have experienced scenarios where the evaluability assessment alone was sufficient to provide the organisation with the information it wanted.

During the evaluability assessment, it is often common to explore the existing sources of data related to the intervention. It may not always be necessary to collect all the information directly from your participants, as data may already be collected which you could use. Thinking about intervention processes and outputs, you might already collect data on the number of participants in the intervention, or how people heard about your intervention. Especially now that devices like phones and tablets are being used so much, these might already be collecting valuable data. The term 'digital exhaust' has been coined to describe the trail of data left behind by most online transactions. While these might not provide your final outcome data, they can provide useful insights about intervention processes. We will go on to cover some of the qualities you might want in a dataset for some of the different evaluation methods.

Ogilvie et al. (2011) proposed five further questions which should be considered as part of the evaluability assessment of complex public health interventions:

- 'Where is a particular intervention situated in the evolutionary flowchart [logic model] of an overall intervention program?'
- 'How will an evaluative study of this intervention affect policy decisions?'
- 'What are the plausible sizes and distribution of the intervention's hypothesized impacts?'
- 'How will the findings of an evaluative study add value to the existing scientific evidence?'
- 'Is it practicable to evaluate the intervention in the time available?'

These questions broaden the perspective of the evaluability assessment to consider the policy landscape and relate to research funders. Adding the economic aspect can help us consider not only whether the intervention worked, but also what contribution the intervention makes. Is that contribution significant enough to merit much wider implementation of the intervention or is the intervention sufficient for the current circumstances? Sometimes an intervention that works for your community is sufficient, especially if its costs can be covered, whilst at other times we are seeking to develop interventions that work for whole regions or countries.

Leviton et al. (2010) described four benefits of conducting an evaluability assessment. First, the exact approach you take to the evaluability assessment will depend on your circumstances, the time you have available and the scope of your intervention. New methods are also likely to be developed for conducting an evaluability assessment. But regardless of this, an evaluability assessment should result in greater engagement with, and commitment to, the evaluation. Particularly, for external evaluation, you don't want people to get the impression that the evaluation is judging them, so greater transparency will make sure there is a shared understanding of the process. Second, the process of the evaluability assessment will help to manage expectations of the evaluation, by making sure these have been agreed before the evaluation commences. Third, the additional time spent refining the programme theory or logic model can improve understanding of the intervention which will help to meaningfully interpret the findings; we will discuss this more in later sections. All of this will lead, fourth, to a better evaluation and is part of the ongoing process of co-production in intervention development.

WHO CONDUCTS THE EVALUATION?

There is one final question to consider before moving onto how to conduct the evaluation. Table 9.1, taken from Naidoo and Wills (2009), outlines the pros and cons of getting someone external (outsider) to conduct the evaluation or conducting it yourself (insider). While getting someone outside your organisation to conduct the evaluation should mean that you don't need to understand all the fine detail of how the evaluation is conducted, the next section provides useful insights that will help you to have informed discussions with those conducting the evaluation. The previous questions and evaluability assessment will ensure that your evaluation meets your needs.

Table 9.1   The pros and cons of having an evaluation conducted by an insider or an outsider (adapted from Naidoo and Wills, 2009)

	Insider evaluation	Outsider evaluation
Pros	Knows project background	Unbiased attitude
	Cheaper	Research expertise
	Acceptable to everyone	Fresh perspective
Cons	Too involved in project	Expensive
	No/limited research expertise	May appear threatening
	Biased to prove success	Unfamiliar with project

Activity 9.2

What, who, when and where to evaluate the 20mph limits?

We don't have information about what Stephanie's intent was for implementing 20mph limits, but these could have included reducing car accidents, congestion, pollution or increasing public transport use or cycling. Consider what other intentions Stephanie might have had for introducing 20mph. This information might have been available in Stephanie's campaign material. For each of the possible outcomes of 20mph limits, describe:

- What you would want to evaluate?
- Who would be the participants in the evaluation?
- When to evaluate it?
- Where to conduct the evaluation?

Consider if the year since implementation of the 20mph limits is sufficient for the evaluation Stephanie wants to undertake. Which stakeholders might Stephanie want to engage in an evaluability assessment? Do you think these stakeholders will agree on what the 20mph limits were intended to achieve, and how would be best to evaluate them?

CONDUCTING AN EVALUATION

There are a lot of evaluation study designs such as the randomised controlled trial, realist evaluation, stepped-wedge or natural experimental approaches listed in the introduction to this chapter (Sanson-Fisher et al., 2014). However, each of these designs is seeking to answer the same set of questions (Sanson-Fisher et al., 2014):

- Has change occurred?
- Did the change occur as the result of the intervention?
- Is the degree of change significant?

Each evaluation study design has strengths and weaknesses when it comes to answering these questions (Sanson-Fisher et al., 2014). There is a subsequent question to ask if the answer to the three questions is 'no', 'if not, why not?', which designs like realist evaluation are designed to answer. The intervention might have worked for some participants and not others, or some components of the intervention might not have worked as expected. These are really valuable insights as we can learn a lot from why an intervention does not work that might prevent us repeating any mistakes. In this section, we explore how the ideas around causality, systems and complexity, introduced in Chapter 3, are applied in practice to answer the three questions above. Before we start on the questions, it is

Knowledge link: This topic is also covered in Chapter 3

important to make sure you understand the difference between the similar sounding but distinct concepts of effect, effectiveness and efficacy (see box on Concept summary). We believe that most of the readers of this book will be interested in establishing the impact of their intervention in practice. So, our evaluations will be seeking to determine effectiveness, with all the complexity this brings. It can also be important to consider whether the effect and efficacy have been established.

Concept summary

effect, efficacy and effectiveness

While these three words are similar, they have important distinctions when it comes to evaluating an intervention. Archibald Cochrane (1909–88), after whom the Cochrane Collaboration (www.cochrane.org) is named, clarified the following distinctions in 1972 (Cochrane, 1972):

- Effect, as in cause and effect. For example, insulin causes glucose to be taken up from the blood stream into the tissues.
- Efficacy, does it work (under ideal circumstances)? For example, does injecting a type 1 diabetic with insulin reduce blood glucose?
- Effectiveness, does it work in the real world? For example, does giving a type 1 diabetic an insulin pen reduce the need for medical attention and enable them to return to a more normal way of life?

Has change occurred?

This relates back to the questions about what to evaluate and when to evaluate it. Some outcomes take much longer to change than others. Think about physical activity and weight – it can take weeks or months for someone's weight to change as a result of their exercise regimen. So, you might be tempted to evaluate the change in physical activity rather than weight. However, someone might adopt a new exercise plan for a week, but then their circumstances change so they cannot maintain the new regimen. Depending on when you measure physical activity, you might reach different conclusions about whether the intervention worked. Physical activity and weight can change over time, but there are other outcomes like taking an exam or developing a disease that only happen once in a lifetime, so the change needs to be examined at the group rather than individual level. In summary, while this question might seem quite simple, what change might look like for your selected evaluation requires some consideration and review of the literature to find out how the outcome is distributed in the population and how it changes. This can be more complicated for subjective outcomes like feelings, emotions and perceptions – even if you ask someone about how happy your intervention made them in an interview, how do you compare two people's reported level of happiness? But the simplest consideration, in terms of establishing whether a change has occurred, is to measure your outcome at least once before and once after the intervention to detect any change. One measurement before (baseline) and one after (follow-up) can be sufficient for designs like a randomised controlled trial, whereas the natural experimental approaches often need multiple pre- and post-intervention measures (Craig et al., 2011; Sanson-Fisher et al., 2014). Even if you only have one baseline measurement of the outcome, it can be useful to collect multiple follow-up measurements to determine if initially change has occurred, and subsequently whether the change has persisted or was just a novelty effect.

Did the change occur as the result of the intervention?

This is the most complicated of the three questions, especially within complex systems. The fictitious evaluation and intervention in Chapter 3 highlighted the importance of control groups, Hawthorn/observer and placebo effects, contamination and randomisation in deriving a definitive answer to the question 'Did the change occur as a result of the intervention?' Evaluation study design can be categorised into three groups: experimental, quasi-experimental and non-experimental. Over the next three subsections, the most common study designs within each group will be briefly introduced, explaining under what circumstances they can be used. For each group of designs, we also discuss the extent to which they address whether the intervention caused the observed change.

Knowledge link: This topic is also covered in Chapter 3

Experimental evaluation designs

In this group are the designs in which receipt of the intervention is conducted experimentally with random allocation and controls. Randomisation ensures that any differences between those receiving the intervention and the control group are due to chance and therefore any differences in the outcome after the intervention can be attributed to the intervention. The most basic experimental evaluation design is the 'randomised controlled trial', where individuals are randomised to receive the intervention or control. If your intervention is delivered to groups of people such as hospital wards, schools or neighbourhoods then you can conduct a 'cluster randomised controlled trial', where the groups of people are randomised to receive the intervention or control. As you would be comparing groups of people within a cluster randomised controlled trial, you need more participants in the study. If your intervention eventually needs to be given to everyone, but you don't have to give it to everyone at the same time, there is a design called a 'stepped wedge'.

Like the cluster randomised controlled trial, groups of people are randomised within this design, but they are randomised into an order in which they will receive the intervention. You measure the outcomes across all the groups before the intervention starts being rolled out, then the first group or groups start receiving the intervention. During this period, the other groups are acting as the control. Weeks or months later, the next group or groups start receiving the intervention, becoming part of the intervention group while the others remain the control group. This continues in steps until all the groups are receiving the intervention but you have collected data from randomised groups to assess the changes in outcomes attributable to the intervention. The stepped wedge design is useful to consider if your intervention requires a lot of resources to set up but then keeps running, and those who set up in one site can move on to setting it up in the next site.

These designs are all described as prospective, that is, you have to start them before the intervention begins and follow up on participants into the future. Where necessary, you need to consider contamination and choose sites or groups for the intervention where any contamination is unlikely. The Hawthorn/observer and placebo effects are common in the experimental designs and need to be considered, otherwise these designs offer the best chance to detect a change attributable to the intervention as you have most control and can ensure that control groups, Hawthorn/observer and placebo effects, contamination and randomisation can be considered. McCambridge et al. (2013) discuss some of the limitations of randomisation, which has practical and ethical considerations.

Quasi-experimental evaluation designs

When it is not possible to randomise people to receive the intervention or control, there is a group of designs called the quasi-experimental designs. If the intervention is a policy change, it might not be possible to introduce randomisation, or the intervention might already be being implemented. The quasi-experimental designs are mostly retrospective, in that they look back on an intervention that has already been implemented, which means that the data used in them have to have already been collected. As you are designing your own intervention using the 6SQuID process, it is less likely that you will be looking to use a quasi-experimental design. One quasi-experimental design makes use of Mendelian randomisation in genetics or other near random processes such as deciding which hospital to go to when you live equidistant between two. These approaches are called 'instrumental variable' (Craig et al., 2011). The other quasi-randomised approach is called 'regression discontinuity' and can be used when receipt of the intervention depends on meeting some measured criteria (e.g. means testing) (Craig et al., 2011). For example, if you needed to have a specific systolic blood pressure to receive an intervention, there is measurement error related to the variation in your blood pressure, the accuracy of the measurement device and the skill of the person undertaking the measurement. So, for those people whose systolic blood pressure is close to the cut point (just above or below), you could consider them randomised to the intervention. These are sometimes called natural experimental approaches as the randomisation has occurred naturally and not been manufactured as in the experimental evaluation designs.

As the designs include a form of randomisation and control groups, they can detect changes attributable to the intervention. By making use of data that has already been collected, these designs are less vulnerable to the Hawthorn/observer and placebo effects. However, the circumstances in which a quasi-experimental study is feasible are quite complicated and rare, meaning we suggest seeking expert advice if you believe a quasi-experimental evaluation is appropriate.

Non-experimental evaluation designs

When it is not possible to randomise receipt of the intervention and there is no randomisation process occurring naturally, differences between the people receiving the intervention or control make it difficult to know if any change detected can be attributed to the intervention. The simplest option is to collect outcome data before and after the intervention in what is called a 'before and after' or 'pre-post' study design. However, if you can still collect data on a control group, it helps give a sense of how the outcome might change without the intervention. You can calculate a difference-in-differences by comparing the difference in outcome from pre- to post-intervention between the groups. When the outcome you are interested in is regularly collected in something like administrative data, an 'interrupted time series' design compares the time series of the outcome before and after the intervention. Again, a difference-in-differences can be calculated when an interrupted time series study includes a control time series. When you have multiple interrupted time series, for example an intervention being deployed across multiple hospitals, the design is called a 'multiple baseline' study, which, much like the stepped-wedge design, can compare periods when one hospital is implementing the intervention and another is not, as intervention and control.

The two major limitations of these designs that prevent them from being used to definitively identify the attributable effect of an intervention are changes over time and differences between the intervention and control groups. Using control groups and time series as described helps to account for any changes that would have happened over time anyway (known as secular trend). Matching can be used to try to account for differences in participants in the control and intervention groups. For each person in the intervention group, you recruit a similar person for the control group, and you might match them in terms of gender, age, health state, and so on. Ideally, you want to match them in relation to any characteristics that might influence their likelihood to achieve the outcome, and this can be quite tricky, which is why randomisation is so useful. The non-experimental designs are mostly used prospectively, but some options like interrupted time series can be used retrospectively if sufficient data are available.

Sanson-Fisher et al. (2014) and Craig et al. (2011) describe these common evaluation designs in more detail, including how to choose between them and their strengths and limitations. While each of these designs has been discussed in relation to quantitative outcomes, qualitative data collection can and should be part of any evaluation. Quantitative data might tell you whether the intervention worked, but it is qualitative data that will tell you how it worked and help you understand why it might not have worked. We will discuss a final set of considerations to ensure your evaluation is ethical and impartial in the next section. The concepts of **bias**, **validity** and **reliability**, which are important when conducting an evaluation, are summarised in the concept summary box.

Concept summary
bias, validity and reliability

These are three important and related concepts to understand when planning an evaluation:

- Bias is any systematic error introduced into data collection and analysis by selecting or encouraging one outcome or answer over others. There are many, many types and details can be found in the Catalogue of Bias (https://catalogofbias.org).
- Validity is the extent to which the evaluation undertaken and the findings from it are accurate and reflect the truth. We try to minimise and avoid bias to ensure that what we do is valid. There are three types of validity to consider:
  - Construct validity – is the underlying theory valid?
  - Internal validity – have any biases been minimised or accounted for, especially in relation to the research methods and data collection?
  - External validity – can the results be generalised?
- Reliability relates to whether, if the methods were repeated, the same results and conclusions would be reached.

Is the degree of change significant?

Finally, all the work you have undertaken applying 6SQuID was probably to ensure that you make an important improvement in the lives of your participants. You want to make a significant change and you want your evaluation to detect that change – we call this the 'effect size'. The work undertaken to understand whether a change has occurred will have given you an insight into how the outcome naturally varies, so you are normally looking for a larger change. But beyond this data-based approach, you would want to know what represents a meaningful or clinical effect size. You could design an evaluation which detected someone smoking one fewer cigarette in their lifetime, but would that make a clinical or meaningful impact on their risk of lung cancer? Sample size calculations undertaken by a statistician are used to work out how many people you need to include in an evaluation to detect the desired effect size. Ideally, all these factors need to have been considered before the evaluation begins and potentially when the intervention is being developed, so that you know how many people need to take part in the intervention to undertake a valid evaluation.

ENSURING YOUR EVALUATION IS IMPARTIAL AND ETHICAL

It is important that not only is the intervention ethical (e.g. The Nuffield Intervention Ladder, Nuffield Council on Bioethics, 2007), the evaluation also needs to be ethical and impartial. The evaluation should not cause any harm (*non-maleficence*), should strive to do good (*beneficence*), treat people fairly (*justice*) and respect their *autonomy*. Ensuring the evaluation is ethical will also help it to be impartial. The standard ethical considerations around competence and consent apply, but briefly discussed below are some additional considerations for evaluation.

Knowledge link: This topic is also covered in Chapters 2, 6 and 7

We have previously mentioned that it is no longer considered ethical to use placebos in evaluations. If someone has the need for an intervention, such as being a smoker, it is not ethical to give them a treatment which is not intended to be beneficial. Subsequently, we often compare a new intervention against the 'gold standard' intervention or usual practice. The evaluation seeks to determine if the intervention is equally as effective as, or more effective than, current practice. If you were a doctor whose patient was in a trial, but you strongly believed that the new treatment was better than the old treatment, would it be ethical to leave the decision for which treatment they received down to chance? This is the effect of randomisation, where you are required to believe that both intervention and control are effective; this is called *equipoise*, which is a balance of forces or interests. Alongside the challenges of randomising allocation of the intervention, maintaining the randomisation and the costs of doing this, equipoise is an important requirement in order to conduct a randomised evaluation. If you have spent all the effort required to follow 6SQuID, might you believe that your new intervention is better than what is already on offer? Subsequently, we are often undertaking evaluations in circumstances which won't permit a randomised controlled trial, and therefore it is even more important to strive to conduct an impartial and rigorous evaluation.

Knowledge link: This topic is also covered in Chapter 3

If your evaluation is taking a qualitative approach or using a questionnaire, it is important that the questions are impartial or unbiased. Looking back at the concept summary box, you can see that this means ensuring that you don't influence people to answer in a specific way with the question wording or response options.

- Instead of asking: 'How much more confident were you after the workshop – A little/ Somewhat/A lot?'

    o   Try: 'Compared to the beginning of the workshop, at the end of the workshop was your confidence – A lot worse/A little worse/About the same/A little better/A lot better?'

It is also important to keep the questions as simple as possible to ensure that anyone reading the question will interpret it similarly. In particular, you should try to only ask about one issue (construct) per question.

- Instead of asking: 'Did you have more confidence and energy after the workshop? Yes or No.'

    o   Try: 'Did you have more confidence after the workshop? Yes or No', and 'Did you have more energy after the workshop? Yes or No'.

Be careful not to be judgemental in how questions are asked or phrased. It is most valuable for you to know people's honest opinions, so you don't want them feeling shamed into specific answers. This is known as social desirability bias, where people will often try to give you the answer they think you want, so it is important to make it clear that all responses are valuable. These considerations are really important to help you identify the possible harms as well as the benefits of the intervention.

Fortunately, questionnaires have already been developed and validated on all sorts of topics, and it would be best to use one of these if they exist. Online searching or consulting experts can help you identify appropriate questionnaires. Be aware that there is a fee for using some questionnaires. The questions you use should be accessible to your participants, with special consideration needed when your participants are children or people with additional needs (vulnerable adults). Moreover, even sticking with written questions and responses can exclude people who have limited literacy or language skills. Therefore, visual methods using images or spoken surveys might be more accessible. There are approaches like photovoice and timelining that can be used to elicit valuable information from people of all abilities.

Finally, there are multiple ways in which an evaluation can do harm. As mentioned previously, there is the obvious risk of harm from specific data-collection techniques like taking blood samples, but even questionnaires can cause harm. Imagine if you had answered a series of questions which reminded you of being harassed in the past, or questions about depression that made you negatively re-evaluate your life. It might be necessary to ask these questions, but you need to plan how participants can be supported or signposted to services should the questions raise issues for them. Any information or data your participants choose to share with you reflects a privileged relationship. It is important to respect that privilege and to store, analyse and dispose of the data accordingly. Imagine how hurt you might feel if you found out your newsagent had told everyone what magazines you buy, or if a sentence out of context from a phone call was published. The General Data Protection Regulations in Europe (and other similar policies) exist to set a legal framework around the appropriate use of data, however we should go above and beyond these to protect the participants in our evaluations.

The process of getting approval for the study from the relevant ethical review boards (e.g. health services, university) will help to ensure the project is ethical and impartial.

SUMMARY

In this chapter, we have worked through the questions you need to consider when planning an evaluation: who, what, when, where, why and how. Evaluability assessment has been introduced as a method for answering these questions in a way that engages all the relevant stakeholders to manage expectations and deliver a better and more informative evaluation. The evaluation designs that can help you establish the effect of your intervention have been described. We have described the need to conduct your evaluation ethically and impartially, mentioning the specific factors that need to be considered to achieve this. Much like intervention development, it is clear that evaluation is complicated, requiring significant preparation time and skills. Therefore, to conclude this chapter we would encourage you to see the evaluation as a team effort, like the intervention itself. You may need to seek advice and support with the evaluation, however you should now be better informed about the decisions which need to be taken to conduct a rigorous evaluation.

FURTHER READING

Beaton, M., Craig, P., Katikireddi, S. V., Jepson, R., and Williams, A. (2014) *Evaluability Assessment of Free School Meals for All Children in P1 to P3*. Edinburgh: NHS Scotland.

Brunner, R., Craig, P., and Watson, N. (2019) 'Evaluability assessment: an application in a complex community improvement setting', *Evaluation*, 25 (3): 349–65. doi:10.1177/1356389019852126

Craig, P., Doi, L., and Tirman, L. (2018) *Scotland's Baby Box: Evaluability Assessment*. www.gov.scot/publications/evaluability-assessment-scotlands-baby-box-report-scottish-government

REFERENCES

Belford, M., Robertson, T., and Jepson, R. (2017) 'Using evaluability assessment to assess local community development health programmes: a Scottish case-study', *BMC Medical Research Methodology*, 17 (1): 70. doi:10.1186/s12874-017-0334-4

Cochrane, A. L. (1972) *Effectiveness and Efficiency: Random Reflections on Health Services*. London: Nuffield Provincial Hospitals Trust. www.nuffieldtrust.org.uk/sites/files/nuffield/publication/Effectiveness_and_Efficiency.pdf (accessed 11 June 2020).

Craig, P., Cooper, C., Gunnell, D., Haw, S., Lawson, K., Macintyre, S., Ogilvie, D., Petticrew, M., Reeves, B., Sutton, M., and Thompson, S. (2011) *Using Natural Experiments to Evaluate Population Health Interventions: Guidance for Producers and Users of Evidence*.

London: Medical Research Council. www.mrc.ac.uk/documents/pdf/natural-experiments-guidance (accessed 11 June 2020).

Drummond, M. F., Sculpher, M. J., Claxton, K., Stoddart, G. L., and Torrance, G. W. (2015) *Methods for the Economic Evaluation of Health Care Programmes*, 4th edn. Oxford: Oxford University Press.

Leviton, L. C., Khan, L. K., Rog, D., Dawkins, N., and Cotton, D. (2010) 'Evaluability assessment to improve public health policies, programs, and practices', *Annual Review of Public Health*, 31: 213–33.

McCambridge, J., Kypri, K., and Elbourne, D. (2013) 'In randomization we trust? There are overlooked problems in experimenting with people in behavioral intervention trials', *Journal of Clinical Epidemiology*, 67 (3): 247–53.

Naidoo, J., and Wills, J. (2009) *Foundations for Health Promotion*, 3rd edn. Oxford: Bailliere Tindall.

Nuffield Council on Bioethics (2007) *Public Health: Ethical Issues*. London: Nuffield Council on Bioethics. http://nuffieldbioethics.org/wp-content/uploads/2014/07/Public-health-ethical-issues.pdf (accessed 13 January 2021).

Ogilvie, D., Cummins, S., Petticrew, M., White, M., Jones, A., and Wheeler, K. (2011) 'Assessing the evaluability of complex public health interventions: five questions for researchers, funders, and policymakers', *Milbank Quarterly*, 89 (2): 206–25.

Sanson-Fisher, R. W., D'Este, C. A., Carey, M. L., Noble, N., and Paul, C. L. (2014) 'Evaluation of systems-oriented public health interventions: alternative research designs', *Annual Review of Public Health*, 35: 9–27.

Wholey, J. S. (1979) *Evaluation: Promise and Performance*. Washington, DC: Urban Institute.

ACTIVITY ANSWERS

Activity 9.1: Why, and for whom, does Stephanie want to evaluate the 20mph limits?

Figure 9.1 gives a few examples.

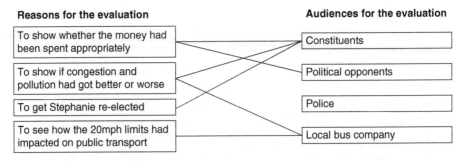

Figure 9.1   Why and for whom does Stephanie want to evaluate the 20mph limits?

Activity 9.2: What, who, when and where to evaluate the 20mph limits?

Table 9.2   What, who, when and where to evaluate the 20mph limits?

	Pollution	Cycling
What?	Motor exhaust fumes and other pollutants such as carbon dioxide or particulate matter	Number of journeys made by bike, change in mode of travel from car to bike
Who?	Probably not any specific individual, but specific places in Edinburgh	People who live and work in the city and can commute by bike
When?	Can be measured from the day the speed limits change	Might not change immediately, so you would want to delay collecting this data, and you would want to make sure any change was not a novelty effect, so you might want to collect data for months or years
Where?	You might pick locations in the city known to have pollution problems	People might fill out surveys on their phones, or there might be automatic cyclist counters, maybe even mobile phone fitness apps

- *Is one year long enough?* It looks like one year would be enough to assess changes in pollution or cycling, but maybe for an outcome like collisions you might need to look at a few years of data as the outcome is fairly rare.
- *Stakeholders for the evaluability assessment* – health service representative, cycling groups, other local politicians and policy makers, public transport organisations, representatives of local schools, local residents, local business owners, etc.
- *Do you think these stakeholders will agree on what the 20mph limits were intended to achieve, and how would be best to evaluate them?* Why might they disagree?

10
CASE STUDIES

Learning objectives

By the end of this chapter, you will understand how 6SQUID has been applied:

- To different problems
- In different settings
- In different ways.

The case studies presented will stimulate your ideas and creativity in relation to how to apply the framework to your own intervention.

INTRODUCTION

By this point, you should be familiar with the 6SQuID steps and feel comfortable enough to apply them to a problem of your choice. Throughout this book, we have used case studies to illustrate specific steps or component parts of steps. This chapter presents case studies outlining the process of 6SQUID (from steps 1–6) in its entirety and is an opportunity to further consolidate your learning and understanding of the key principles and steps outlined in this book. We invited four teams to contribute a case study illustrating how they have used 6SQuID in their own practice. These case studies demonstrate how the steps have been applied in different contexts, illustrating its flexibility and, ultimately, its usefulness. The four case studies outlined in the remainder of this chapter focus on the problems of:

1. HIV and treatment adherence in South Africa;
2. Sedentary behaviour in contact centres in the UK;
3. Gestational diabetes in the UK;
4. Injuries and deaths in forestry work in an indigenous population in New Zealand.

Since some of these case studies are recent, some have not yet moved onto Step 6: Evaluation. In those case studies, they describe what they will be doing in the future.

CASE STUDY 1. HIV INFECTION AND TREATMENT ADHERENCE

The team developing this intervention worked closely with stakeholders at all stages of the development process. Stakeholders included those familiar with the context in which the intervention was to be delivered: the non-governmental organisations that would implement the intervention; government officials and academics.

Choosing a problem to address

This intervention focused on the problem of adherence to antiretroviral treatment (ART) amongst people living with HIV in South Africa (Masquillier et al., 2020). In South Africa, an estimated 7.5 million members of the population are living with HIV (UNAIDS, 2021). In 2016, a Universal Test and Treatment programme was implemented to ensure access to ART for all people who test HIV-positive. However, prevention and treatment adherence issues remain. Incidence of new infections remains high and only 64% of those persons living with HIV receiving treatment have undetectable viral loads (i.e. suppressed virus) (UNAIDS, 2021).

What has been done before to address the problem?

Large-scale roll-out of ART began in 2003. This programme is central to bringing an end to the HIV epidemic in South Africa. However, issues related to the supply and retention of health professionals has been one of the most serious obstacles to the sustainable implementation of the treatment plan. In search of the mobilisation of new human resources for health, tasks have shifted to community health workers (CHWs) and people living with HIV themselves. However, given the current treatment and prevention challenges, there is a need for new sustainable interventions that draw upon non-health service resources to reduce HIV infections and to support those persons living with HIV to manage their condition and treatments successfully. Such interventions could focus on the untapped potential of the household, which would provide much needed support to a strained Universal Test and Treat programme.

Understanding the causes of the problem

To develop an intervention, an understanding of the causes of the problem is necessary. The team conducted a literature review and qualitative research to identify contextual factors in which these HIV-related challenges unfold. A conceptual model was developed to illustrate these factors, how they relate to one another and how they ultimately contribute to the problem, as shown in Figure 10.1.

The conceptual model of factors illustrated that barriers to treatment adherence and preventive behaviour exist at the community, household and individual levels. The team concluded that the social context of the household provides an important potential source of support for treatment adherence. Successful management of HIV is not only dependent on the individual but also on whether their household provides an environment that is conducive to a lifestyle that promotes health. This occurs within the wider backdrop of various community-level influences. Within this context, the team argues that intervention is needed to increase 'HIV competency' within households (Masquillier et al., 2015).

Identifying modifiable factors

Two modifiable factors were selected for intervention: equipping individual person living with HIV to become an HIV-competent individual; and communication at household level, in particular issues around the disclosure and sharing of HIV-related knowledge. The team's research indicated that communication was a core part of what they refer to as an 'HIV-competent household'. The team theorised that both increasing knowledge and fostering safe communication would likely lead to the promotion

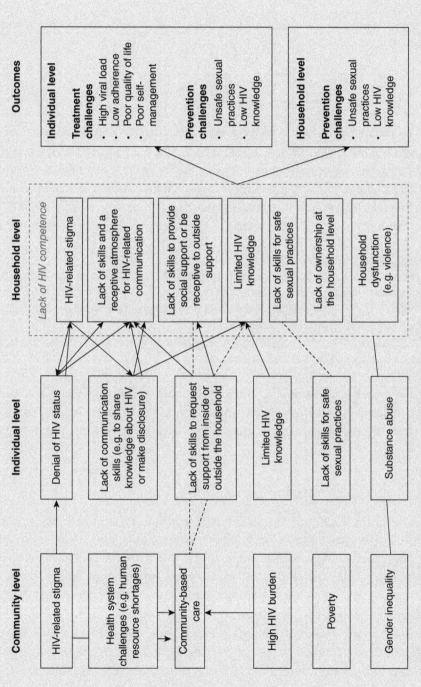

Figure 10.1 Factors contributing to HIV treatment and prevention challenges

Source: Masquillier et al. (2020) (CC BY)

of preventive practices, and support for PLWH in the household in terms of treatment adherence.

Developing a theory of change

Based on research at early phases of the work, the team developed what they called the 'Positive Communication Process' (P²CP) model. This model represents a mechanism of change to trigger the expected outcomes. The model describes the four steps required to build 'HIV competency' in the household, in which a household member is encouraged to disclose their HIV status to a confidante (i.e. a trusted household member) with whom he/she can then build 'HIV competency' in the household. The four steps are as follows:

1. Recognising the reality of HIV in the household
2. Disclosure of HIV to at least one other household member, ideally someone who is influential within the house
3. Person living with HIV and their confidante become 'change agents' through sufficient knowledge and communication skills training
4. Change agents become 'household advisors' by sharing knowledge on treatment, support and prevention to the wider household.

The team proposed that this would result in a household that increases and maintains treatment adherence and reduces likelihood of infection of other household members. The relationship between theory of change and outcomes is shown in Figure 10.2.

Developing a theory of action

Each level of the P²CP model was operationalised into specific activities, as shown in Figure 10.3. The intervention is delivered by a community health worker and consists of seven sessions of one-hour duration across the four P²CP steps and is shown in Figure 10.3. The intervention aims to facilitate 'HIV competence' by fostering positive communication and sharing of HIV knowledge. Visits one and two are geared towards the individual level, specifically developing the self-management skills of the persons living with HIV. Visits three and four are focused on the interpersonal level, containing activities to improve communication in addition to exercises focused around HIV status disclosure. Visits five and six are focused at the household level and contain activities to stimulate knowledge and support in addition to fostering ownership. Thinking about sustainability, the intervention developers geared the seventh and final session towards maintenance of the skills learned, specifically focusing on planning for long-term support.

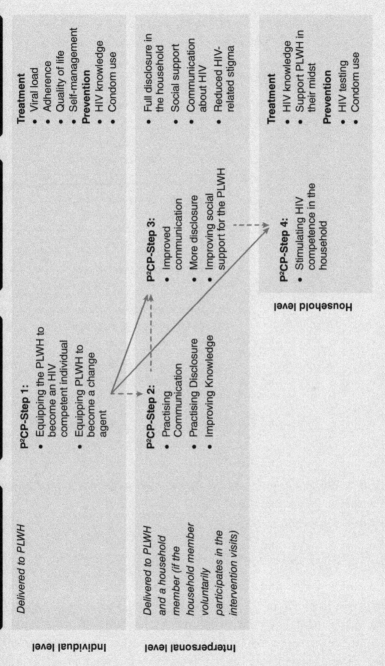

Figure 10.2 Theory of change for household HIV treatment and prevention intervention

Source: Masquillier et al. (2020) (CC BY)

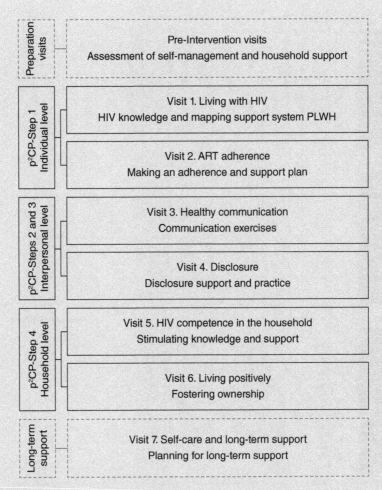

Figure 10.3 Session overview of the Sinako intervention based on the 'Positive Communication Process' model

Source: Masquillier et al. (2020) (CC BY)

Testing and adapting on a small scale

The intervention was piloted with two patients who underwent all seven sessions. These sessions were recorded and analysed by the research team, with a view to revising the intervention content if necessary. Additionally, the team held debriefing sessions with the community health workers delivering the intervention to gain specific insight into what worked well and what might need to be tweaked before full implementation. The findings indicated that the intervention content itself did not require to be tweaked. However, the piloting flagged an issue with the rigidity of the intervention visiting schedule. The team tweaked the intervention to be more flexible as a result of this finding.

Debriefing sessions with community health workers delivering the intervention identified that they felt further training on delivery was necessary. The team therefore extended the training period in response to this.

Due to the COVID-19 pandemic, the intervention had to be halted after being implemented for four months. At that time, 152 people living with HIV had started the intervention. The community health workers who implemented the intervention were interviewed to learn from their implementation experience. More attention in the training was requested related to the communication skills of the community health workers in their interaction with the persons living with HIV, and treatment fidelity should be assessed in a different way. The lessons from these first few months of implementation were taken into account when restarting the intervention after the COVID-19 measures allowed doing so.

Lessons from using 6SQuID in the real world

In this case study, the 6SQUID model proved useful in guiding the research team through all the necessary steps to develop a sound intervention. The sixth and last step of the 6SQUID framework is the implementation and evaluation of the intervention in a real-world setting. However, this implementation study encountered a couple of unexpected delays, stemming from policy changes in the field, as well as the COVID-19 pandemic.

CASE STUDY 2. SEDENTARY BEHAVIOUR IN CONTACT CENTRES
Choosing a problem to address

The Stand Up For Health project aims to address the issue of sedentary behaviour in contact centres. Sedentary behaviour is a serious occupational health hazard, linked with an increased risk of type 2 diabetes, cardiovascular disease, musculoskeletal issues and poor mental wellbeing. Contact centres are associated with higher levels of sedentary behaviour than other office-based work. Contact centre staff spend 95% of their shift sitting, and one in four members of contact centre staff regularly experience musculoskeletal problems, with 22.4% of sick days lost to such problems. Given the lack of policies from authoritative bodies that are specific to sedentary behaviour, it is imperative that preventative approaches are implemented, underscoring the need to develop interventions to reduce sedentary behaviour in contact centres.

What has been done before to address the problem?

Contact centres are settings with complex processes at play. Reducing sedentary behaviour requires an intervention which accounts for the various interacting levels and factors perpetuating a sedentary environment. Only a few studies have taken a multilevel approach to reducing sedentary behaviour in contact centres. One study explored factors influencing physical activity and sedentary behaviour among call agents (Morris et al., 2018). They reported that employees describe contact centres as stressful work environments due to low workplace autonomy, performance monitoring and commission-based salary systems. Moreover, there are organisational pressures to maintain high levels of productivity and meet targets, and leaders and managers often perceive that health and physical activity programmes reduce the agents' call-making time and lead to productivity losses (Renton et al., 2011).

Studies have reported a low level of knowledge of guidelines and recommendations relating to sedentary behaviour and physical activity, and a lack of awareness about sedentary behaviour as a risk factor for poor health among contact centre agents, team leaders and senior staff (Coenen et al., 2017; Morris et al., 2018).

Understanding the causes of the problem

Researchers from the Scottish Collaboration for Public Health Research and Policy (University of Edinburgh) worked with staff and managers at the Ipsos Mori contact centre to understand the causes of sedentary behaviour in contact centres. This stage of intervention development was informed by a literature review, a survey and focus groups with staff members of Ipsos Mori. Individual, organisational, social and environmental themes were identified (see Table 10.1).

Table 10.1 Factors causing sedentary behaviour in the workplace

Level	Factors causing sedentary behaviour
Individual	• Stress • Lack of motivation • Lack of knowledge about sedentary behaviour • Pre-existing health problems • Perception of having no control of health at work • Fatigue
Social	• Co-worker behaviour • Workplace pressures that foster sitting • Workplace culture around break taking • Norm of communicating through electronic means

Level	Factors causing sedentary behaviour
Environmental	• Ergonomic set-up • Feeling tied to their desk • A perceived need to be seated while working
Organisational	• Nature of contact centre work • Strict work schedule, such as having limited breaks • Heavy workload and pressure to be profitable • High staff turnover • Support from management

Identifying modifiable and non-modifiable factors

Factors identified from the literature review, survey results and focus groups with staff members were then categorised as modifiable and non-modifiable and presented as a fishbone diagram. This is shown in Figure 10.4.

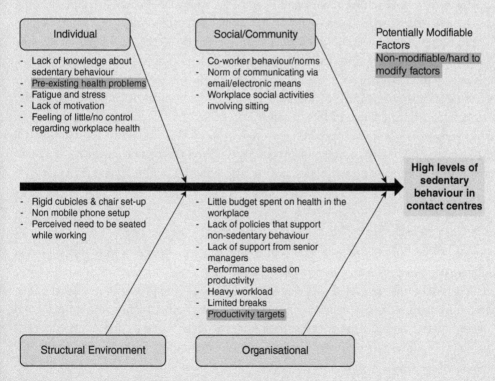

Figure 10.4 Stand Up For Health: fishbone diagram

Understanding the available assets and resources

The Stand Up For Health team worked with contact centre managers to understand context (e.g. centre layout, work-time flexibility, shift patterns) and resource availability (budget, space, online material, equipment, staff members with physical activity or other expertise). They used a resource assessment template to map out the assets and resources for the centre.

Developing a theory of change

The theory of change underpinning Stand Up For Health is shown in Figure 10.6. Note that the theory of change occurs at different levels of change from individual behaviour to organisational-level change. The theory of change was informed by a mixture of both existing and working theory. For example, the developers proposed that goal-setting and the provision of incentives (the mechanism of change) will increase motivation, which will in turn lead to sitting less and moving more at work, which will in turn lead to a number of benefits for staff, including increased focus and concentration and fitness, in addition to wider benefits for the centre. The mechanism of change in this instance is informed by goal-setting theory and operant learning theory. Similarly, intervention developers propose that the recognition and implementation of changes which support staff to sit less and move more will lead to Stand Up For Health becoming part of working routine. The intervention developers hypothesise that this will lead directly to staff feeling valued and to a happier, healthier workplace in the longer term. It will also directly lead to staff sitting less and moving more at work and a number of long-term outcomes. The mechanism of change in this instance is informed by stakeholder views as to how best to trigger this outcomes chain, i.e. working theory. It is important to note that, for the Stand Up For Health programme, it is fidelity to the theory of change that is important, rather than being prescriptive about specific activities that bring about change.

Developing a theory of action

A workshop was conducted at the Ipsos Mori contact centre to inform the development of a theory of action, i.e. to operationalise the theory of change. The workshop was designed to include activities associated with one of the four levels from the socio-ecological framework leading to sedentary behaviour (individual, social/community, environmental and organisational), and incorporated feedback from the focus group sessions with staff. Staff members were invited to join, try out equipment (e.g. standing desk riser, treadmill, desk bike, exercise bands, stepper machines) and participate in mindfulness activities like colouring, jigsaws, and so on. The research team crafted a prioritisation exercise with three

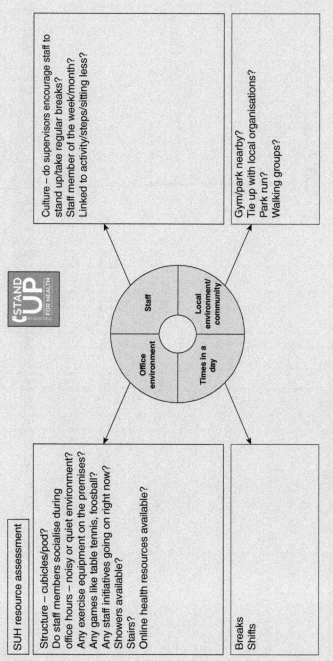

SUH resource assessment

Structure – cubicles/pod?
Do staff members socialise during
office hours – noisy or quiet environment?
Any exercise equipment on the premises?
Any games like table tennis, foosball?
Any staff initiatives going on right now?
Showers available?
Stairs?
Online health resources available?

Breaks
Shifts

Office
environment

Staff

Times in a
day

Local
environment/
community

Culture – do supervisors encourage staff to
stand up/take regular breaks?
Staff member of the week/month?
Linked to activity/steps/sitting less?

Gym/park nearby?
Tie up with local organisations?
Park run?
Walking groups?

Figure 10.5 Stand Up For Health: resource assessment

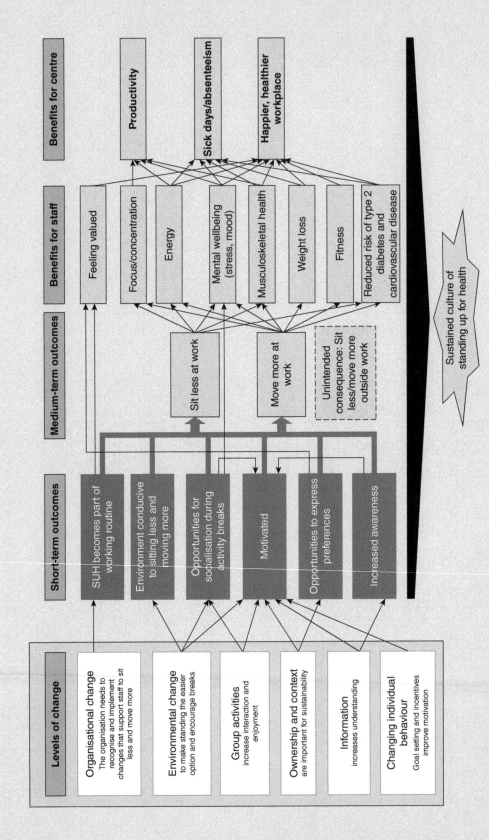

Figure 10.6 Stand Up For Health: theory of change

flipcharts illustrating the individual, social and environmental activities suggested by researchers (Figure 10.4). Staff at the workshop rated the equipment and individual and social activities by placing sticky dots next to the names of activities on flipcharts. Findings from the prioritisation exercise were used to decide which activities would be implemented. The Stand Up For Health team worked with contact centre managers to understand the context of the contact centre (e.g. centre layout, work-time flexibility, budget and resources available) using a resource assessment template (see Figure 10.5).

After the workshop, the Stand Up For Health team developed an action plan for the centre and discussed the implementation of activities with centre managers. Activities at each level of the theory of change were considered and discussed, in the context of resource availability, shift times and budget. The Stand Up For Health team encouraged the adoption of at least one activity from each level of the theory of change. A 'SMART' approach (specific, measurable, achievable, realistic (or relevant) and time-bound (or timely)) was adopted to enhance the success of implementation.

Testing and adapting on a small scale

Having developed the programme theory in a pilot centre, the next step was to test and refine the intervention. An NIHR-funded feasibility trial (www.fundingawards.nihr.ac.uk/award/17/149/19) is under way to evaluate the intervention delivery and implementation, and to procure preliminary estimates of effectiveness, the details of which are shown in Table 10.2. The team held two workshops. In the initial workshop, staff tried out various equipment and activities and participated in the prioritisation exercise. The Stand Up For Health team also lent several pieces of equipment (exercise bike, stepper, twisting disks, mini table tennis, mini golf, etc.) to the centres, keeping in mind environmental factors and staff preferences. The Stand Up For Health team then worked with the centre coordinator to develop an action plan specific to the centre. The team came back to the centre for a second workshop after three months, where they spoke to the staff about implementation, likes and dislikes, so that the action plan could be further refined.

The Stand Up For Health project team completed all intervention delivery and data collection activities in February 2020, but was forced to abandon in-person visits to contact centres due to the COVID-19 pandemic. However, the team was able to remotely deliver a modified programme consisting of sessions with staff, providing suggestions to sit less and move more, and a step-count challenge, in addition to activities specified locally by the contact centres themselves. The team is in the process of analysing study data. Despite the disruptions, results show that Stand Up For Health was successful in creating change at the individual, social, organisational and environmental levels. The study fostered a strong sense of ownership among staff members and increased knowledge and awareness about sedentary behaviour and physical activity. The pandemic has given rise

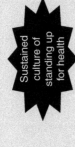

Sustained culture of standing up for health

Individual behaviour
- Motivational techniques – goal setting (weight loss, fitness, steps)
- Desk-based stretches
- Token system (where individuals get tokens for meeting targets and work towards centre goals)

Information
- Website
- Delivery of messages

Ownership and context
- Initial event prioritising outcomes
- SUH committee includes staff from all levels
- Making sure all activities are fit for purpose

Group activities
- Charity run/walks
- Walking/running groups
- Team-based activities
- Competitions
- Yoga/Tai Chi classes
- Bingo

Environmental change
- Equipment from SUH team
- Placement of equipment and designated SUH spaces
- Changes to desk structure

Key Element

Organisational change
- SUH committe
- Action plan
- Included in induction
- Changes to working routine
- Supervisor buy-in

Levels of change

Changing individual behaviour
Goal setting and incentives improve motivation

Information
increases understanding

Ownership and context
are important for sustainability

Group activities
increase interaction and enjoyment

Envi ronmental change
to make standing the easier option and encourage breaks

Organisational change
The organisation recognises and implements changes that support staff to sit less and move more

Figure 10.7 Stand Up For Health: theory of action

Table 10.2   Stand Up For Health: feasibility study details

Title	Stand Up for Health: A feasibility cluster randomised controlled trial (RCT) of a theory-based intervention to reduce sedentary behaviour in contact centres
Study Design	Feasibility cluster randomised controlled trial with a process evaluation component
Number of centres recruited and location	11 centres across the UK (London, Newcastle, Durham, Edinburgh)
Study outcomes	Primary outcome: Objectively measured sedentary time in the workplace, using an activPAL™ device Secondary outcomes: • Subjective measures of sedentary time in the workplace • Objectively measured total sedentary time and physical activity • Productivity • Mental wellbeing • Musculoskeletal health

to a hybrid mode of working, combining office and home working, and the study will use data from the process evaluation and consults to refine Stand Up For Health programme theory to reflect this change.

Lessons from using 6SQuID in the real world

6SQuID provided a strong theory-based framework to develop the Stand Up For Health programme. Over the course of intervention development, the importance of co-production and considering the context became evident. Each contact centre is unique, with its own internal and external systems, and working with stakeholders and staff to consider organisational culture and environment was vital to successful implementation. This allowed for the implementation of a range of activities, enhancing the appeal and inclusiveness of the programme. Communication and coordination with various teams in the centre, such as health and safety, and centre managers, were critical. The focus on theory of change rather than specific activities meant the programme was flexible and could be adapted to real-world issues such as the COVID-19 pandemic.

Another learning point was that change may be a slow process, so it is important to acknowledge and celebrate small changes and wins. The project team also noted that certain levels of intervention can be more resistant to change. In the Stand Up For Health study, it was difficult to implement changes at the organisational level. Perhaps a lesson is to recognise that some change mechanisms are easy to implement and efficacious in the short to medium term, while others may take longer and require greater effort, and to develop a strategy to address this.

CASE STUDY 3. PHYSICAL ACTIVITY IN WOMEN AT HIGH RISK OF TYPE 2 DIABETES

Choosing a problem to address

Gestational diabetes is a type of diabetes that onsets during pregnancy for women and typically resolves once the baby is born. Mothers who have gestational diabetes may have to change their diet and exercise pattern when diagnosed to protect their health and the health of their unborn child. This is because unmanaged gestational diabetes can result in complications during pregnancy and delivery. Once they give birth, their diabetes typically resolves immediately, and they can return to their 'normal' eating habits and way of life. However, they have an up to ten times higher risk of getting type 2 diabetes in the future, in comparison to women who have had children but not had gestational diabetes.

Women with a history of gestational diabetes can reduce their risk of getting type 2 diabetes by eating well, exercising and managing their stress. However, research suggests that many women with previous gestational diabetes do not meet the levels of physical activity recommended in guidelines. This problem was the focus of a doctoral research project at the University of Edinburgh. The present case study sets out the steps taken to develop a physical activity intervention for women with previous gestational diabetes, using steps 1 through 4 of 6SQuID, as seen in Figure 10.8.

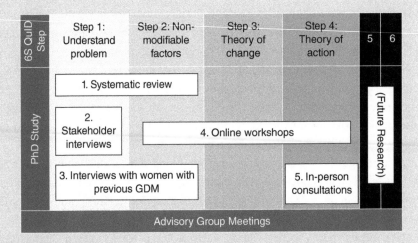

Figure 10.8 Overview of gestational diabetes intervention development

What has been done before to address the problem?

Physical inactivity is a difficult problem to change in any population. Few interventions have resulted in sustained increase in physical activity. A mixed methods synthesis identified many factors that women said were important to them that were not addressed by any interventions and included: lack of time/energy to be more active, feeling guilty, putting off health behaviour change, healthcare professional support, feeling helpless about type 2 diabetes onset, being a healthy role model and issues with breastfeeding. Walking, pedometer use and education about type 2 diabetes risk were mismatches, meaning women said it was important but interventions that addressed these factors did not appear more effective. Interventions that addressed factors such as access to childcare, social and community support and culturally sensitive engagement seemed more effective than interventions that did not include these. Overall, this review informed what had been done before and what should be addressed in the future.

Understanding the causes of the problem

Three different types of data were used in this step, as seen in Figure 10.8: a systematic review, interviews with key stakeholders and then interviews with women with current and previous gestational diabetes. The intention was to understand the problem from different perspectives and using different types of evidence – an international level from the systematic review, a community level by speaking to key stakeholders and an individual level from the in-person interviews.

After conducting, analysing and synthesising the qualitative data from the three studies, a synthesised fishbone diagram (see Figure 10.9) was developed in order to understand the multitude of contributing factors to physical inactivity. It's clear from this fishbone diagram that there are many barriers to physical activity in the lives of these women, spread across all levels of the social determinants of health model.

Identifying modifiable and non-modifiable factors

The factors from the fishbone diagram were then sorted into modifiable, potentially modifiable and non-modifiable factors. This was based on the interviews with the women, talking to the participant advisory group and the results of the systematic review.

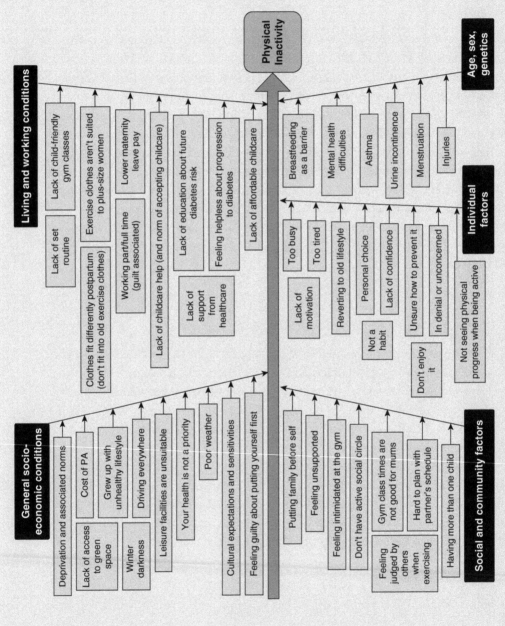

Figure 10.9 The contributory factors to physical inactivity for women with a history of gestational diabetes

Table 10.3 Sorting the fishbone diagram into modifiable, potentially modifiable and non-modifiable factors

Modifiable	Potentially modifiable	Non-modifiable
Lack of understanding of future risk of diabetes	Not seeing physical progress when being active	Deprivation and associated norms
Cost of physical activity	Clothes fit differently postpartum	Lack of set routine
Urine incontinence		GDM is a transient condition
Don't enjoy activity	Exercise clothes aren't suited to plus-size women	Having more than one child
Feeling judged by others when exercising	Lack of continuity of care	Lack of access to green space
Putting family before self	Hard to plan with partner's schedule	Grew up with unhealthy lifestyle
Mental health difficulties	Lack of childcare help (and norm of accepting childcare)	Winter darkness
Your health is not a priority		Driving everywhere
Personal choice to be inactive	In denial or unconcerned	Leisure facilities are unsuitable
Physical activity is not a habit	Don't have active social circle, partner, family	Lack of child-friendly gym classes
Feeling helpless about progression to diabetes	Reverting to old lifestyle	Menstruation
Feeling unsupported	Lack of affordable childcare	Injuries
Lack of education about future diabetes risk	Too tired	Working part/full time (guilt associated)
Lack of motivation		Gym class times are not good for mums
Too busy		Lower maternity leave pay
Feeling guilty about putting yourself first		Asthma
		Cultural expectations and sensitivities
		Poor weather
		Breastfeeding as a barrier

The most prevalent barrier to physical activity that women identified was that they are not a priority in their own lives – everything else comes before them. They do not feel it is feasible nor acceptable to take time for themselves until everyone else has been taken care of – both a never-ending task and a gendered one. Many of the barriers identified in the fishbone diagram were related to this key factor, and as such it was theorised that addressing this factor would have far-reaching improvements in women's lives – including increasing their physical activity behaviour.

Understanding the available assets and resources

To understand what local physical activity programmes were available and if they were suitable for women with previous gestational diabetes, local physical activity professionals (e.g. people who ran physical activity programmes at community leisure centres) were interviewed about the programmes they ran. Overall, no interventions were found that were perfectly suited to women with previous gestational diabetes – either the age range was not suitable, or the focus of the programme was inappropriate, or there was an absence of suitable childcare. However, two key stakeholders were identified in this stage of the research that were key assets in the development of the subsequent intervention.

Developing a theory of change

To develop a theory of change and action, group consensus was needed with the stakeholders. After speaking with a lay advisory group and discussing various online or telephone options, a secret Facebook group was decided to be the tool of choice to co-produce a theory of change and action. Over 15 days, 21 women with a history of gestational diabetes took part in developing a theory of change and action, based on the results of the previous three studies.

To address the factor of prioritising activity in their own lives, the primary theory of change is that improvements in mindfulness and self-compassion (treating yourself as you would a close friend) will result in improved self-prioritisation and, subsequently, causal factors to physical inactivity such as stress, anxiety, feeling guilty about putting yourself first, low confidence and poor body image, will diminish.

Other key theories of change that underpinned the theory of action were as follows:

- Focusing on the mental and physical health benefits of physical activity, rather than weight loss, will result in more sustainable physical activity behaviour.
- Having access to a safe and supportive online environment with similar women will improve the sense of social support and problem-solving ability within their lives.
- Motherhood-specific and functional exercises will increase motivation for and enjoyment of physical activity.

Developing a theory of action

Following the development of the theory of action, the intervention was named Moving Forward with Gestational Diabetes. The Moving Forward programme aims to address the theories of change through three phases, in which the first phase is a mindful self-compassion programme that elicits key outcomes to make physical activity more feasible in women's lives. The next phase introduces physical activity through short, functional home exercise videos and the final phase ensures sustainability. Underlying all of these phases is social support within a secret Facebook group. The logic model in Figure 10.10 provides a detailed overview of the programme components and key outcomes.

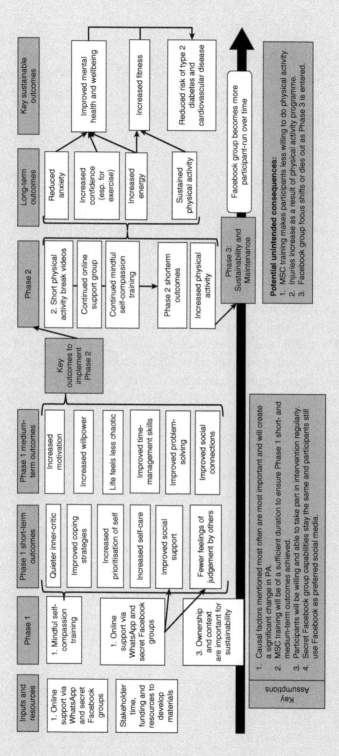

Figure 10.10 The Moving Forward with Gestational Diabetes logic model

The next stage of 6SQuID would be to test and adapt on a small scale – this could be done in a small-scale feasibility test where participants would try out the different components, provide qualitative feedback and then revise as needed until few changes are suggested after each round. Then a more rigorous evaluation could take place before wider implementation.

Lessons from using 6SQuID in the real world

The 6SQuID framework was an excellent starting point for a doctoral research project, as it allowed for in-depth exploration of the causes of the problem and how it should best be addressed. The iterative nature of the steps was highlighted as a lesson learned. In the PhD there wasn't one study for Step 1, another for Step 2, and so on. At the start of the PhD research, the 6SQuID framework appeared to be in discrete steps, with each piece of research encompassing one step of the framework, resulting in a neat and tidy group of studies. It was quickly realised that this isn't always the case. A framework such as 6SQuID, being a broadly applicable tool for public health, social care and even policy development, is meant to structure your thinking about a problem and its solutions. It is not a tick-box exercise nor is it a definitive manual to follow line by line.

At times, there was a tendency for the team to try to skip ahead to the theory of action, as participants and stakeholders would become interested in novel intervention ideas and start making suggestions. It's important to note them, but not follow the line of thinking too far when you aren't at that stage of the intervention development process yet. This is where intervention development studies can be led astray, by jumping to the theory of action prior to being explicit about the most important and modifiable factors and then developing the theory of change. In addition, Step 3 in this PhD felt conceptually the most complex of the 6SQuID steps – describing the change mechanism sometimes seemed obvious or exceedingly difficult – and at times it felt easier to move ahead to the theory of action rather than wrestle with the concept of a theory of change.

CASE STUDY 4. MANAIASAFE FORESTRY SCHOOL

Whakatauki

I orea te tuatara ka patu ki waho

A problem is solved by continuing to find solutions

In the Māori worldview, a manaia is a guardian, caring for the safety and wellbeing of people. From October 2018 to February 2019, a 20-week ManaiaSAFE Forestry School (MFS) pilot programme ran in Tairawhiti (Gisborne) on the east coast of Te Ika a Maui (the North Island) of Aotearoa New Zealand. The MFS aim was 'to deliver an innovative, safety based, real world, forestry harvesting learning experience and environment, engaging young people on an educational and career pathway to high quality jobs and skills'.

An independent evaluation of the pilot programme used the Six Steps of Quality Intervention Development (6SQuID) model (Wilkie, 2018). 6SQuID notes that:

> Improving the effectiveness of ... interventions relies as much on the attention paid to their design and feasibility as to their evaluation. Yet, compared to the vast literature on how to evaluate interventions, there is little to guide researchers or practitioners on how best to develop such interventions in practical, logical, evidence based ways to maximise likely effectiveness ... If each of these steps is carefully addressed, better use will be made of scarce public resources by avoiding the costly evaluation, or implementation, of unpromising interventions. (Wight et al., 2016)

What is the problem?

Research by WorkSafe, Aotearoa New Zealand's primary workplace health and safety regulator, found that low-quality training was an issue in forestry:

> The external training in the [forestry] industry is viewed as being of low quality and difficult to access, particularly the off-site entry-level courses, which are seen as not providing a realistic understanding of the forestry working environment and subsequently those who graduate have no real understanding of the workplace they encounter. (WorkSafe New Zealand, 2017)

A primary motivation behind the development of the ManaiaSAFE Forestry School was the unacceptable level of preventable deaths in the local forests that impacted heavily on the *whānau* (families) and communities. At the time of the MFS pilot, the rates of fatalities and serious injury in the forests nationwide, although reducing, were unacceptably high. In the year to 21 December 2018, five forestry fatalities were reported (WorkSafe New Zealand, 2019). Three of the forestry deaths directly impacted the MFS communities.

What has been done before to address the problem?

Nigel Udy, Head of School of Primary Industries of the Eastern Institute of Technology in Gisborne, that partnered with MFS, described the problem of meeting the demand for forestry training in the region:

Forestry is one of the largest primary sectors in the Tairāwhiti region and so it really is a no-brainer that we should be trying to assist and help support, service, the forestry sector, for identifying and training people for that industry. Over the last few years 2015–17 we have tried, and I would have to say failed in meeting that need and that demand of the sector.

By the training that we had done we had found it difficult to recruit and retain appropriate students. We found it difficult for drug related issues for people that we had on the training programme as well as for the forestry industry. We finished up that style of delivery at the beginning of 2018 but still knowing that there was a great need.

Manaiasafe have come in with a concept of supplying and delivering in a much more sup-ported manner to students and thinking about them from a holistic perspective. Certainly, the achievements are much better than what we achieved by ourselves previously and there is no question about that.

We know if I am a School in Primary Industries for tertiary education and I'm in the Tairāwhiti region and I'm not doing anything in Forestry there is this great gaping hole. I can use any excuses like we tried, and nobody wanted to do the training … I always feel there is this emptiness there if we have got a very significant forestry Primary Sector, and we aren't doing anything in it. (Wilkie, 2019c)

In the scoping for the pilot evaluation, Henry Koia, the MFS managing director and project manager, used the 6SQuID model to describe the issues and development of the MFS training, a selection of which are presented here.

Understanding the causes of the problem

New Zealand's long-standing forestry skills shortage is stifling industry growth and increasing risk to health and safety inside the forest gate. Several factors contribute to this problem:

- Recruitment challenges with barriers to entry to work in forestry that is broadly per-ceived as a dangerous industry, including financial challenges and public perceptions.
- Lack of effective training for new entrants to a 'work-ready' standard before they walk on to a commercial forest operation. The current on-the-job approach where responsibility for training delivery is left to the commercial operators does not work well.
- Limited effective competencies development of those already in the forestry workforce.

Identifying modifiable and non-modifiable factors

From the MFS's view, each of the factors listed above is modifiable and has scope for great change:

- Recruitment challenges could be lifted by a change to the entry choices currently on offer to prospective new entrants. One option would be a pathway set up for new foresters to receive quality training and qualifications, to level 3 of the National Qualifications Framework, in a controlled environment, before walking on to a commercial forest operation. This pathway would also need to offer financial support to meet living costs while in training.
- By changing how the industry defines 'work ready' in the forestry context to be 'having the knowledge, skills, experience, and values that a contractor is able to use immediately in their daily work'. Then to change the way training is delivered to bring new entrants up to 'work-ready' standards.
- Offering changes to the way in-work competence development is delivered so that those already working in the industry have access to quality training and national certification, that takes place outside of a commercial production environment.

Developing a theory of change

The proposed mechanism for change on the three issues identified above is the new Manaia Workforce Management Model, designed by Manaia Safety Systems Limited for the forest industry workforce. With ongoing research and evaluation, including skills demand and supply forecasting, the Manaia Workforce Management Model would deliver the following four critical outcomes:

1. New entrants recruited
2. Work-ready training and qualifications delivered
3. In-work competence developed
4. Worker inflow and outflow managed, concerning skills retention and replacement.

Developing a theory of action

The ManaiaSAFE Forestry School (MFS) offered a new forestry training model designed to help address the forestry skills shortage by focusing on delivering the four critical outcomes of the Manaia Workforce Management Model.

The MFS training model offered a pathway into the forestry industry that combined quality training to achieve national qualifications including safety skills. It features a unique forest-based training environment, where learners are mentored under strict supervision by highly experienced bushmen, before moving on to a commercial forest operation. This unique forest-based training environment can be leveraged in many ways to help develop in-work competence across the industry to support better safety and productivity outcomes.

Testing and adapting on a small scale

The ManaiaSAFE Forestry School pilot project was essentially about testing the feasibility of the training model and acquiring critical knowledge through research and evaluation to help predict whether establishing a national network of ManaiaSAFE Forestry Schools was a quality intervention that would benefit Aotearoa New Zealand in the long term.

The MFS pilot put 11 students through a 20-week cable harvesting training programme where graduates could gain the New Zealand Certificate in Forest Harvesting Operations (Level 3) with strands in either tree-felling and quality control, breaking-out cable, or manual processing and quality control. Of those 11, 8 trainees gained certificates and graduated into work in the industry, with some continuing on to higher-level qualifications in forestry.

Collecting sufficient evidence of effectiveness to justify rigorous evaluation/implementation

One major goal of the pilot project was to deliver a high-quality research report on time, on budget and to a standard underpinned by academic rigour to either support or discredit the claim that a national network of ManaiaSAFE Forestry Schools is likely to deliver significant benefits to the forest industry and its supplier network, forest-based communities across the regions, Maori and Pasifika, and the national economy.

The research and evaluation reports were created to determine what, if anything, would eventuate beyond the pilot, including:

- whether government and industry decision makers would have the confidence to partner with MFS for scale-up, to deliver further programmes;
- whether the government would instigate high-level evidence-based policy change (including the training funding) that better delivers skills for the forest industry;
- potential for improvements to productivity and safety that could be achieved in other industries such as horticulture, through applied learning.

Lessons from using 6SQuID in the real world and next steps

In 2019, central government part funded the expansion of the ManaiaSAFE Forestry School into three training sites. Industry partners and income generated from real-world harvesting by MFS crews contributed to the training. In April 2020, COVID-19 closed the gates to all of the forests in Aotearoa and impacted on the commercial viability of the school.

By the end of 2020, Train Me Quality Services, trading as ManaiaSAFE Forestry School, was registered by the New Zealand Qualifications Authority (NZQA) as a Private Training Establishment (PTE) and became eligible for direct government funding for their training programmes.

The resources developed for the pilot evaluation are still in use for self-evaluation and development of the MFS training. More information and updates can be found online:

- 2021 confidence in MFS: Government-funding-boosts-forestry-career-pathways
- YouTube: Manaiasafe videos
- Facebook: www.facebook.com/ManaiasafeForestrySchool
- Website: www.manaiasafe.co.nz

REFERENCES

Coenen, P., Gilson, N., Healy, G. N., Dunstan, D. W., and Straker, L. M. (2017) *Applied Ergonomics*, *60*: 320–33.

Masquillier, C., Wouters, E., Mortelmans, D., and van Wyk, B. (2015) 'On the road to HIV/AIDS competence in the household: building a health-enabling environment for people living with HIV/AIDS', *International Journal of Environmental Research and Public Health*, *12* (3): 3264–92.

Morris, A., Murphy, R., Shepherd, S., and Graves, L. (2018) Multi-stakeholder perspectives of factors that influence contact centre call agents' workplace physical activity and sedentary behaviour. *International Journal of Environmental Research and Public Health*, *15* (7): 1484.

Renton, S., Lightfoot, N. E., and Maar, M. A. (2011) 'Physical activity promotion in call centres: employers' perspectives', *Health Education Research*, *26* (6): 1050–9.

UNAIDS (2021) 'South Africa: HIV and AIDS estimates'. www.unaids.org/en/regions-countries/countries/southafrica.

Wight, D., Wimbush, E., Jepson, R., and Doi, L. (2016) 'Six steps in quality intervention development (6SQuID)', *Journal of Epidemiology and Community Health*, *70*: 520–5.

Wilkie, M. (2018) ManaiaSAFE Forestry School Pilot Evaluation. *Report 1: Scoping and Initial Review.* Gisborne: Train Me Quality Services.

Wilkie, M. (2019a) ManaiaSAFE Forestry School Pilot Evaluation. *Report 2: Kaupapa Māori Social Cost Benefit Analysis.* Gisborne: Train Me Quality Services.

Wilkie, M. (2019b) ManaiaSAFE Forestry School Pilot Evaluation. *Report 3: Pilot Formative Evaluation.* Gisborne: ManaiaSAFE Forestry School.

Wilkie, M. (2019c) *ManaiaSAFE Forestry School Pilot Evaluation.* Gisborne: ManaiaSAFE Forestry School, 29 March.

WorkSafe New Zealand (2017) *Training and Workforce Development in Forestry.* www.worksafe.govt.nz/worksafe/research/research-reports/2016-forestry-research/2016-forestry-research-documents/2016-Forestry-Research-Report-6.pdf

WorkSafe New Zealand (2019) *WorkSafe Fatalities Data.* https://worksafe.govt.nz/data-and-research/ws-data/fatalities

11
CONCLUSION

Learning objectives

By the end of this chapter, you should:

- Understand the importance of practising the 6SQuID steps
- Understand issues that should remain under consideration as you move past the development stage, including fidelity, transferability and sustainability
- Know how to disseminate your findings
- Know how the framework can be used to teach intervention development
- Understand the current state of intervention development and future directions in this field
- Be able to find learning and training resources which may benefit you in your professional development as an intervention developer.

INTRODUCTION

As intervention developers, we strive to create positive and sustainable change. This requires appropriate methods. Such methods should take account of complexity, including the context and systems within which we intend to implement our interventions. Throughout the previous ten chapters, we have aimed to provide you with the understanding and skills necessary to develop such an intervention, with close input from the local community and wider stakeholders. In doing so, we have attempted to shine a spotlight on iterative processes that may not always be immediately apparent and can at first appear somewhat opaque, such as the development of theory of change and theory of action. We have emphasised the central role that co-production should play in ensuring that your intervention is sustainable, acceptable and effective. Working alongside others is a fundamental prerequisite of any intervention operating within an existing system or systems. By drawing out these processes and providing a step-by-step account of the methodologies involved, we believe that we have provided a comprehensive, up-to-date practical guide to intervention development that is useful to anyone working in this field.

APPLYING 6SQuIWD

This book has outlined the 6SQuID steps and underpinning concepts in considerable detail. We have intentionally done this in the spirit of being over-explanatory rather than providing you with too little information. As with the development of all skills, you will improve with practice.

It might be helpful for you to begin trying out some of the steps on a problem or issue in your own life, keeping notes as to which of the steps you find easy or difficult. For example, you could try to develop an intervention to help you manage your work-load better, or spend more time with your family, or increase your own personal sense of wellbeing. The 6SQuID framework is something that you can use for the smallest of problems to the largest. By spending time applying it (or thinking about how to apply it) to your own life, you can start to find out where some of your assumptions lie (e.g. I don't exercise because I don't have time) and how the systems around you impact on the decisions you make. Familiarity with the steps through focusing on something that is close and personal to you will help you to then apply the steps to problems on a larger scale.

The authors of this book and some of our colleagues who use the framework often use the 6SQuID steps in our day-to-day problem solving. We can be heard to say 'Let's 6SQuID it' fairly frequently when a problem is raised, no matter how small. By applying the framework to day-to-day problem solving, you may find that this further consolidates your learning and prepares you for applying it to something larger scale. Another way to practise your understanding is to look at any of the policies and programmes out there, and critically appraise them through a 6SQuID lens. To do this, you would work back-wards from what the policy or programme provides to try to identify the problem it has been created to solve. You may be surprised by how often there has been little thought put into the process or activities being delivered. For those activities that are ineffective, you can begin to understand what makes them ineffective. For example, is it ineffective because there is a far more important causal factor that has not been addressed? Or is it because the 'dose' is too low (e.g. one session of yoga a month for depression) to even expect meaningful change? Or perhaps it is simply not acceptable or relevant for the population group (e.g. a cycling route for people who cannot afford bicycles, or have no place to store them)? By applying the framework in these ways, intervention development will soon become second nature.

Intervention development is an art as well as a science. You should let yourself and others enjoy the process, encouraging creativity and innovation within the process. Do not be scared to try various activities out. If they fail, explore why. Sometimes activities fail, not because they are ineffective, but because an assumption has been made that has not been identified and mitigated against. We believe that 6SQuID offers a flexible framework within which to experiment with different approaches. We embrace exploration, practice and innovation as core features of the intervention development journey. This has the bonus of strengthening bonds between team members as you combine efforts and enjoy the journey towards a well-developed intervention.

ISSUES FOR CONSIDERATION AS YOU MOVE PAST THE DEVELOPMENT STAGE

Implementation of your intervention in the coming weeks and months should be at the forefront of your consideration. Throughout this book, we have advocated for an approach of co-production. This brings numerous benefits as outlined previously. A co-produced intervention should result in an intervention that is sufficiently embedded in the systems in which it is to be implemented. This should reduce the likelihood of implementation issues further down the line, since those implementing the intervention should have been actively involved in planning how it will work in practice. However, it is still good practice to be collecting data as to how well your intervention is being implemented. This can be done by liaising closely with those delivering your intervention, collecting data on aspects of delivery (either through surveys or qualitative interviews, or informal conversations if resources are limited). The success of your intervention is dependent, not only on its content, but also on how well it is delivered. A well-designed intervention may not work well to achieve its intended outcomes if it is poorly delivered.

Knowledge link: This topic is also covered in Chapter 2

The issue of intervention fidelity was highlighted in relation to steps 3, 4 and 5. Fidelity is defined as the degree to which interventions are implemented as intended. Fidelity is closely linked to adaptation, with the potential for both positive and negative effects if interventions are tweaked (Perez et al., 2016). We have argued in this book that overemphasis on fidelity to specific intervention activities (i.e. theory of action) may harm intervention outcomes in some cases. This is because adaptations may be necessary to ensure that the intervention can operate within its intended context. Those who are involved in implementing interventions should be able to adapt content to ensure

Knowledge link: This topic is also covered in Chapters 6, 7 and 8

Knowledge link:
This topic is
also covered in
Chapter 8

that it is appropriate to contexts and systems. We have argued that theoretical fidelity – adherence to the 'essence' of the intervention or the theory of change – is likely far more appropriate to the implementation of complex interventions. This means that the theory of action (i.e. the activities) may change according to the context and constraints of the system, but the theory of change remains the same. The challenge for those implementing such interventions is to find the appropriate balance between adaptation and fidelity to theory of change, such that the intervention retains its effectiveness.

The concept of fidelity to the theory of change is linked to that of transferability: the extent to which your intervention (and its component activities) can be implemented in different contexts and population groups. An intervention to improve cardiovascular health might have a healthy eating component and a physical activity component. Both components will contain activities aimed towards improving cardiovascular health. This may include written materials and workshop materials. The specifics of the intervention may look quite different depending on the context in which it is being delivered. Fundamentally, you have seen in this book that interventions target causes to create change. The causes of a problem may differ depending on context. For example, the accessibility of healthy food and venues for physical activity may be a cause of poor cardiovascular health in one context but not another. If you are thinking of transferring your intervention to another context, you should think very carefully as to whether the causes underpinning that intervention and all its subsequent content are also causes in relation to the new context.

Even if the underpinning causes are similar, adaptations may still be necessary. Such adaptations should strive to retain fidelity to theory of change. If our cardiovascular health intervention in the previous paragraph was developed in the United States, tweaks to content would be required prior to implementation elsewhere. These tweaks might include changes to the language used in any written materials or changes to workshop materials to make them less US-centric, or to the format of the intervention itself – for instance, number of sessions, length of workshops – depending on the new context in which it is being implemented. It may be the case that entire components of the intervention are just not relevant in other contexts – in this case, an entirely new intervention may be required. It is extremely rare to find an intervention that is truly transferable without some adaptation. However, such adaptations can usually be done without deviating from the underpinning theory of change.

Knowledge link:
This topic is
also covered in
Chapters 2, 3
and 7

The period following intervention development should also involve a continued consideration of the sustainability of the intervention. When we create an intervention, we want it to be sustainable as well as effective. Sustainability is usually a direct consequence of the extent to which an intervention is embedded within the systems and routines in which it is implemented (Proctor et al., 2011). This is why there is such a focus on sustainability and systems throughout the 6SQuID steps. We highlighted potential harms resulting from poorly thought-out unsustainable interventions. Any potential benefits are likely to fizzle out once an intervention is withdrawn which can affect participants' enthusiasm and morale. The point at which intervention development ends is not clear cut. To increase the likelihood of maintaining sustainability, your intervention should have a mechanism by which further refinements can be made, whether by a nominated champion who is responsible for advocating for the needs of the intervention or ongoing monitoring and further tweaks if necessary (Bodkin and Hakimi, 2020). A healthy and sustainable intervention is one that is not rigid, but dynamic and with scope for further refinements to ensure it is achieving the intended outcomes.

DISSEMINATION

Dissemination refers to the process of sharing your findings with wider stakeholders, members of the population including those who participated in your intervention and those who may benefit from applying some of the findings in their own practice, such as colleagues, policy makers and wider practitioners. It is considered good practice to disseminate as widely as possible, since your findings may contain learning that could be useful for others. Perhaps they are working in the same field and looking to develop an intervention to tackle a similar problem. By sharing your findings, you are contributing to a body of knowledge that could be applied by others. It is important to note that negative findings have equal value to positive findings – knowing that something has not worked and had to be changed could be useful for others developing similar interventions.

The TiDieR-PHP reporting guideline for population health and policy interventions advises that intervention developers report the following characteristics of the process: the rationale behind the intervention including how intervention activities are linked to the expected effects on causal factors and outcomes, what materials are used, how the intervention was planned and delivered, who provided it, where it was provided, when and how often it was provided, and aspects of its delivery, such as how well it was delivered (Campbell et al., 2018). The idea is to be as detailed as possible in your reporting such that the intervention can be replicated elsewhere. Of course, the level of detail you report can be highly dependent on the method of dissemination. For example, if your team is planning to submit a paper for publication in an academic journal, you may find that there are numerous space constraints in terms of word count. Most academic journals allow for authors to submit supplementary material which can be helpful. We typically find that intervention dissemination involves multiple formats. Typically, there is a detailed report in which sufficient information of the type outlined in the TiDieR-PHP reporting guideline can be reported. This is usually accompanied by other outputs.

Table 11.1 Methods of dissemination

Method	Description
Policy brief	Short in length; typically requested by policy makers; focuses on key findings and their implications for policy and practice
Academic journal paper	Technical account of the development process and outputs; can vary in length but typically short to mid-length; generally insufficient space to be overly detailed although supplementary materials are usually allowed
End of project report	Length can vary; opportunity to go into detail that might not otherwise be appropriate for other formats, e.g. very detailed description of intervention activities; the end of project report is something that should always be written; can be adapted for different audiences
Oral presentation	Limited length; good for brief overviews and take-home points. Can be adapted for different audiences
Social media, e.g. Twitter	Good for engaging a variety of audiences; take-home points most appropriate; should be accessible and avoid technical language
Workshop	Good for engaging stakeholders with findings; feeding back to the target group; can be adapted for different audiences
Media brief	If your work is of interest to local or national media, you may wish to prepare a media brief; these should be very short and punchy accessible summaries of your findings
Creative methods	Good for engaging a variety of audiences; video shorts; cartoons; music, etc.

Table 11.1 outlines some methods of dissemination that you may wish to consider. It is important to agree with your team which outputs and formats would be most useful for them and for your intended audience. For example, there may be policy makers on your team who would appreciate a policy brief. Similarly, there may be community groups involved who would prefer a workshop to engage members of the community. To engage more widely with interested parties, you may choose to utilise social media to share bite-sized take-home points with others who may find the learning to be useful. If your work is of interest to local or national media organisations, you could also consider preparing a short media brief with key take-home points. We have generally found that it is good practice to make your outputs as accessible as possible so that your work can be accessed by a variety of different groups. There is a place for technical reports, but it is essential to also consider other, more accessible dissemination methods.

USING THE FRAMEWORK TO TEACH INTERVENTION DEVELOPMENT

We have applied 6SQuID in various forms of educational contexts over the past seven years. In community settings, we have used either the whole framework or specific steps of the framework as part of workshops to stimulate creative thinking around solutions to various public health problems, in the hope that the methods learned will go on to be applied in practice. We have delivered teaching on the framework as part of the Master's in Public Health curriculum at the University of Edinburgh. This course had a high number of registered students each year and received extremely positive feedback, which we believe indicates a thirst for this type of practical and applied content in a new generation of individuals working in public health and allied fields. We believe this book would make an excellent textbook for any course that focuses on intervention development and fits readily into a ten-week programme. We also believe it would be useful as supplementary reading for courses which cover public health methods more widely.

We have learned much about what seems to work best when teaching the framework. Our teaching philosophy has always been that 6SQuID is taught best when there is sufficient opportunity to engage in group work. This closely simulates intervention development in the real world and gives a flavour of the benefits of this approach to working, in addition to important learning about the types of issues that can arise. We propose that students are split into groups and asked to identify a problem that they will focus on for the remainder of the course. The remainder of subsequent classes focus on each of the 6SQuID steps, with sufficient time set aside at the end of these for practical group work exercises. This process essentially simulates real-world intervention development. If you are thinking of using this book to plan teaching around 6SQuID, we would propose that you be creative in terms of how it can best fit the learning needs of your audience. You can use the activities within this book but we would also recommend that you tweak the content to make it more applicable to your specific context if necessary. In this sense, teaching 6SQUID is a bit like an intervention itself. Example 10.1 nicely illustrates this point by showing how 6SQuID has been creatively adopted into the university teaching curriculum in New Zealand.

Example 10.1

Use of 6SQuID as part of the university teaching curriculum in New Zealand

In New Zealand, the Treaty of Waitangi outlines the relationship between Māori and the Crown. In public health, intervention development cannot be considered without reference to the treaty. As part of a course using 6SQuID to develop interventions, students are asked to consider the framework alongside the treaty. One of the activities asks students to outline the interconnections between treaty and framework. Figure 11.1 shows a diagram produced by Shauni Burke, who undertook the course. She explains the shared respectful foundations which underlie both treaty and framework.

(Continued)

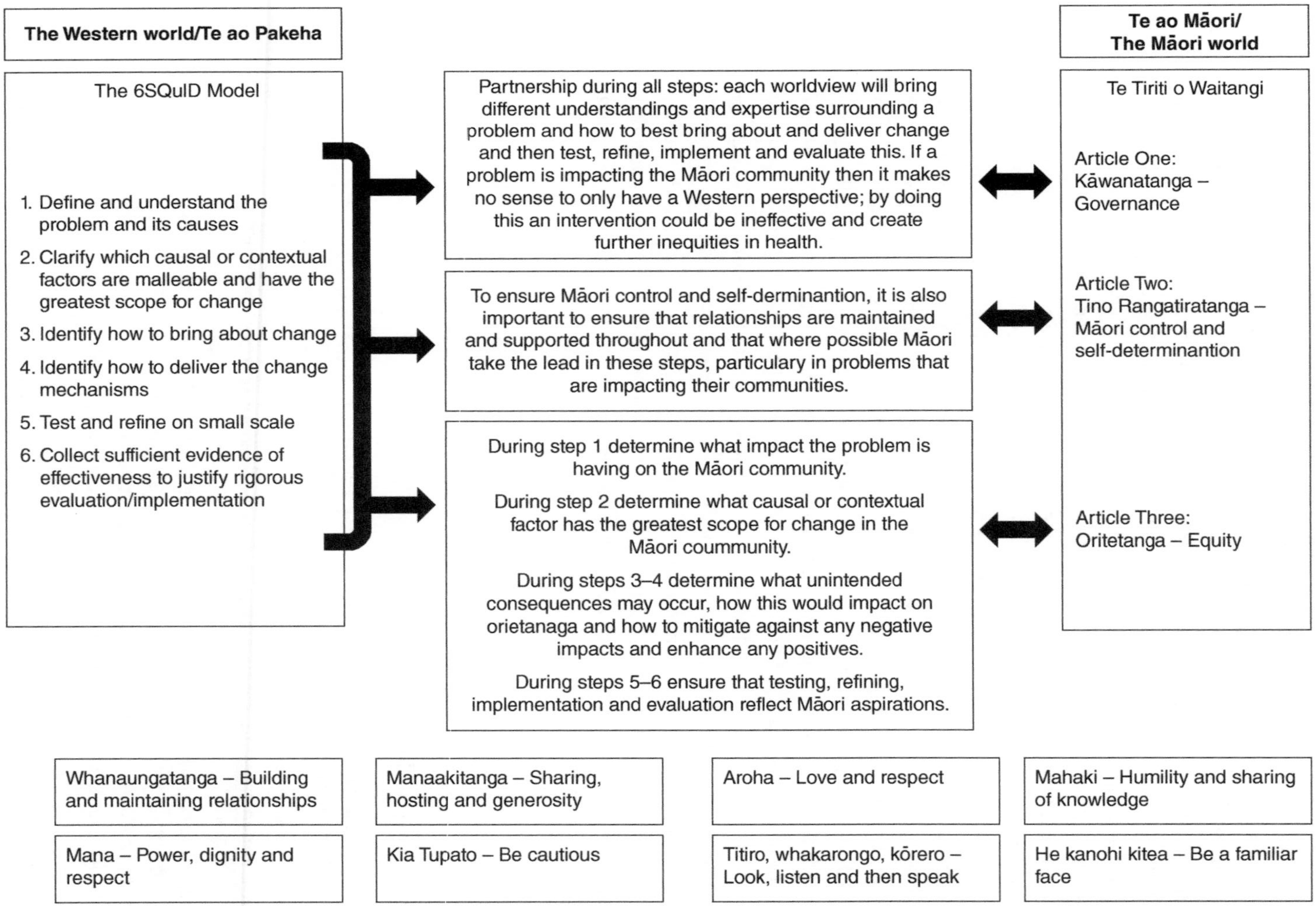

Figure 11.1 Shared respectful foundations

I have put the 6SQuID model in the Western world as this intervention model largely draws from this perspective. I have put te Tiriti o Waitangi in te ao Māori as it is paramount in ensuring that interventions draw from te ao Māori. I have blended these two colours to create a place in the middle that represents a meeting of these two worlds. Underneath this I have placed eight principles outlined by Linda Smith and Fiona Cram (2001) as I believe these are foundational in fostering the interconnection between these two worlds. In the middle I have provided three ways to incorporate Kāwanatanga, Tino Rangatiratanga and Oritetanga into all the steps of the 6SQuID model, however these are just some examples of how they can connect which are coloured by my worldview. Consultation with different communities would likely reveal further ways that te Tiriti o Waitangi and the 6SQuID model can or do interconnect.

FUTURE DIRECTIONS FOR THE FIELD OF PUBLIC HEALTH INTERVENTION DEVELOPMENT

This is a stimulating time to be involved in the field of public health intervention development. Methods in the field have progressed a great deal from didactic intervention development led by a researcher based in a university setting to appreciation of the different types of knowledge and experiences necessary to build an effective and sustainable intervention within what are often multiple different systems. More generally, there is a wider appreciation of the need for and value of considered intervention development. This is perhaps a direct result of the public's exposure to public health interventions on a large scale in response to the coronavirus pandemic. Almost everyone has had an opinion on some of the large-scale interventions implemented across the world which have affected us all in some form or another. We have heard from many colleagues and friends (many of whom do not work in public health) what they think has worked, what hasn't worked, why this might be the case and what might have worked better. This type of thinking is integral to intervention development and we believe that many people are now beginning to recognise that solutions to complex problems must be thoroughly thought through.

There is a growing recognition of the need to co-produce interventions for them to stand the greatest chance of success. However, challenges still exist and need to be overcome for this approach to become commonplace. In their paper examining stakeholders' experiences of the research process in outdoor space and non-communicable disease prevention, Laird et al. (2020) identified challenges to true collaborative working. For example, academic participants in this study expressed concerns about the role of non-academics (defined as practitioners and policy makers) in shaping the research agenda. These concerns feel incredibly outdated, even though this study is only a year old.

Sadly, there are some who believe that they know best and do not see the value of a multi-perspective, cross-disciplinary and cross-sector approach for identifying long-lasting solutions. This way of thinking can be hugely damaging in a team setting and can result in members of the group feeling disenfranchised and undervalued.

We propose that all knowledge and experience are valuable. Co-production provides a method by which to bring disparate but related knowledge and experience together to ensure that an intervention has the best chance of success. All parties involved in the act of intervention share one common goal: to create positive change in the specified outcome. This cannot be achieved without bringing those parties together. It is during these interactions that interventions are shaped for the better.

It is important to view 6SQuID as a dynamic framework which may change as the science of intervention development progresses in the future. We advise against rigidity in its application and encourage you to be flexible and to experiment as you apply it within your own life and practice. 6SQuID should also not be seen as a prescriptive framework, operating in a linear fashion. Intervention development is a very iterative process and what we have found is that intervention developers frequently return to earlier steps as they progress.

CONCLUSION

As human beings, we have been applying solutions to problems since early childhood. Our ability to think through problems and arrive at solutions is a unique part of the human experience. In this sense, we are intervention developers by nature. Much of what we have covered in this book has expanded this problem-solving process to ensure it can be appropriately applied to larger problems in the world. We believe that 6SQuID is rigorous enough to ensure that the intervention produced is acceptable, sustainable and has the best chance of being effective. It is flexible enough to allow for creativity in your approach with the emphasis on iterative development rather than static linear steps. We have positioned co-production as an essential aspect of the intervention development process rather than as an optional extra. Effective teamwork is also necessary, with equal value placed on different types of knowledge and experience. We recognise that people may use this book in different ways and apply it to a whole range of problems. We would be delighted to hear from you as you begin to navigate the process of applying 6SQuID to your own context. Most of all, we hope you enjoy the process as much as we do.

FURTHER LEARNING

As you have seen throughout this book, intervention development involves co-production and teamwork. These are skills that again improve with practice. However, there are a number of free resources that are available online. You may wish to consider learning more about group facilitation. Facilitation refers to the process of effectively working with a group to achieve the agreed outcomes. Facilitation skills are useful for ensuring that all members of your team are able to contribute to the group and these can create a sense of ownership. Free facilitation resources are available online such as those produced by the UK Institute of Cultural Affairs (www.ica-uk.org.uk/facilitation-learning-resources). Similarly, free co-production tools are available that can assist you in ensuring that your intervention is co-produced. The UK third-sector organisation IRISS has produced a free co-production project planner which comes with a number of tools and workbooks (www.iriss.org.uk/resources/tools/co-production-project-planner).

If you are exploring ideas around disseminating your findings, the UK Health Foundation has produced a free toolkit which focuses on planning for impact, communicating your findings and widening impact (www.health.org.uk/publications/communicating-your-research-a-toolkit). These are useful tools which we would encourage you to look at and make use of. You may also find other materials online that can assist with aspects of the intervention development process.

REFERENCES

Bodkin, A., and Hakimi, S. (2020) 'Sustainable by design: a systematic review of factors for health promotion program sustainability', *BMC Public Health*, *20*: 964.

Campbell, M., Katikireddi, S. V., Hoffmann, T., Armstrong, R., Waters, E., and Craig, P. (2018) 'TIDieR-PHP: a reporting guideline for population health and policy interventions', *BMJ*, 16 May; 361: k1079. doi: 10.1136/bmj.k1079. PMID: 29769210; PMCID: PMC5954974.

Laird, Y., Manner, J., Baldwin, L., Hunter, R., McAteer, J., Rodgers, S., Williamson, C., and Jepson, R. (2020) 'Stakeholders' experiences of the public health research process: time to change the system?', *Health Research Policy Systems*, *18*: 83.

Perez, D., Van der Stuyft, P., Zabala, M. C., Castro, M., and Lefevre, P. (2016) 'A modified theoretical framework to assess implementation fidelity of adaptive public health interventions', *Implementation Science*, *11*: 91.

Proctor, E., Silmere, H., Raghavan, R., Hovmand, P., Aarons, G., Bunger, A., Griffey, R., and Hensley, M. (2011) 'Outcomes for implementation research: conceptual distinctions, measurement challenges, and research agenda', *Administration and Policy in Mental Health and Mental Health Services*, *38* (2): 65–76.

Smith, L. T., and Cram, F. (2001) 'Community up model: Māori ethical frameworks'. Available at: www.rangahau.co.nzKnowledge link: This topic is also covered in Chapter 10

GLOSSARY

Term	Definition
Acceptability	The extent to which people delivering or receiving an intervention consider it to be appropriate or acceptable.
Activity/Action	Part of an intervention aimed at reducing a risk factor (or risk factors). An intervention may consist of a single activity (e.g. a mass media campaign) or multiple activities (e.g. 20mph signs, plus educational campaign, plus legal enforcement). See also INTERVENTION and THEORY OF ACTION
Assets	The resources of an individual, community or system that can be utilised to increase the acceptability, sustainability and effectiveness of the intervention.
Assets-based approach	Asset-based approaches emphasise the need to redress the balance between meeting needs and nurturing the strengths and resources of people and communities. They are ways of valuing and building on the skills, successes and strengths of individuals and communities, which focus on the positive capacity of individuals and communities rather than solely on their needs, deficits and problems. These assets can act as the foundation from which to build a positive future. The identification and mobilisation of an individual's or a community's assets can help them overcome some of the challenges they face and create a shared vision and ownership of the intervention.
Bias	Any systematic error introduced into data collection and analysis by selecting or encouraging one outcome or answer over others within an evaluation.
Causal loop diagrams	Diagrams showing the relationships between causal factors and how they operate within a system (or systems).
Causality	Cause is what makes something else happen; effect refers to what results. Cause is the why something happened and effect is the what happened. In intervention development, we often refer to effect as the *outcome* or *outcomes*. See also DETERMINANTS and RISK FACTORS
Change mechanism	A lever which triggers a sequence of outcomes in an outcomes chain.
Co-production	An approach in which researchers, practitioners and the public work together, sharing power and responsibility from the start to the end of the project, including the generation of knowledge.
Complex interventions	May have multiple, interacting components and non-linear causal pathways, with variability in the content, context and mode of delivery, as well as the unpredictability of their effect on outcomes.
Complexity	A state of being complex, confusing or entangled.
Construct	A component part of a theory.
Cost-effectiveness	Whether the intervention can be effective at affordable costs.

Term	Definition
Determinant	A variable associated with an increased risk of an outcome. For example, poverty is a determinant of non-communicable diseases. See also RISK FACTOR
Dissemination	The process of sharing your findings with stakeholders, members of the population including those who participated in your intervention and those who may benefit from applying some of the findings in their own practice.
Distal risk factor	A risk factor that is more distant from the level of the individual and is less modifiable (e.g. poverty) but will result in bigger health impacts. See also PROXIMAL RISK FACTOR
Effectiveness	The impact of an intervention in the real world.
Efficacy	The impact of an intervention under ideal circumstances, such as in a laboratory.
Emergent property	In relation to complex systems, this term describes a behaviour or an outcome of a system that results from relationships within the system. This is difficult to predict based on the components of the system. The property could be positive or negative. For example, we can understand how neurones in the brain transmit information. The fact that this simple process maintains our memories and allows us to dream and imagine is not predictable from the activities of individual neurones.
Ethics	A system of moral principles which we use to guide our decision making as we navigate the process of intervention development.
Evaluability assessment	A pre-evaluation activity designed to maximise the chances that any subsequent evaluation of programmes, practices, or policies will result in useful information.
Evaluation	An assessment, as systematic and impartial as possible, of the effects of an intervention, including effects on outcomes, costs, acceptability and the wider systems in which it is implemented.
Feasibility	Testing whether it is practical to implement the intervention, or collect the data needed for a fuller evaluation.
Feedback, and feedback loops	Describe the relationships between causal factors and other causal factors/outcomes in which the relationship is not linear (e.g. a lack of available healthy food leads to a poor diet). Instead, one factor can influence another. For example, drinking too much caffeine may lead to sleeplessness, and too much sleeplessness may lead to drinking more caffeine.
Fishbone diagram	Also called a cause and effect diagram or Ishikawa diagram. This is a diagram used to visualise the possible causes of a problem and facilitates the sorting of causes into categories.
Grey literature	Any type of literature that is not published in the academic literature. It is usually published by non-research related organisations to share their results for funders, stakeholders and the general public.
Hard to modify risk factor	A risk factor that is difficult but not impossible to change. Examples are poverty and substandard housing.

Term	Definition
Health inequalities	Differences in health outcomes between different groups within the population. Health inequalities have been shown across income, ethnicity, gender, disability, sexual orientation and social class. These factors have also been shown to interact with one another.
Intervention	A *planned action* (or set of actions) that is designed to bring about a *desired change* (of one of more outcomes) in a defined population in order to address a social or health problem. They may be called programmes, policies, services or projects, but their common aim is to 'intervene' in order to have a desired effect.
Intervention development team	A team comprised of a range of stakeholders who will co-develop the intervention.
Logic model	Diagrams showing hypothesised cause and effect relationships between short-, medium- and long-term outcomes.
Meta-analysis	A statistical method of combining data from multiple studies.
Mind-mapping	A diagram to visually organise information. Used to show the relationships between causes of the problem and the problem itself.
Modifiable risk factor	A risk factor that can be reduced to some extent by an intervention. Examples include smoking behaviour, alcohol intake and physical inactivity.
Multi-perspective approach diagrams	Diagrams that enable the visualisation of multiple perspectives. Useful at the beginning of intervention development to define the problem.
Necessary cause	A casual factor without which the effect cannot occur. For example, the lung condition mesothelioma would not occur without the inhalation of asbestos; asbestos is therefore a necessary cause of mesothelioma.
Needs assessment	A method to understand the needs of the population and the type and distribution of health and care services that will bring the greatest benefit.
Non-modifiable factor	A risk factor that is not amenable to change. Examples include age and ethnicity.
Operationalisation	The practical specification of activities employed to activate your underpinning theories of change.
Pilot study	A version of the main study that is run on a small scale to test whether the components of the main study can all work together.
Programme theory	Theory describing how an intervention is expected to trigger a chain of outcomes through specified activities. Consists of a theory of change and a theory of action.
Propensity score matching	An analysis technique whereby you use the observable matching factors within a statistical logistic regression model to find people who have similar propensity to be exposed to the potential cause, but only give one of them the potential cause or only one of them actually was exposed. The use of the propensity scores is intended to account for observed and unobservable factors in the matching, but this does not always seem to work.
Proximal risk factor	A risk factor that is closer to the level of the individual and is therefore more immediately amenable to change (e.g. attitudes and beliefs).
Randomised controlled trial (RCT)	An evaluation study design in which there is a control group who do not receive the active ingredient of the intervention, and individual people are randomised to receive the intervention or control.

Term	Definition
Reliability	Whether, if the methods were repeated, the same results and conclusions would be reached.
Rich pictures	A visual way of building a picture of the collective views and perspectives of those involved. Can be used to define the problem, and to identify the systems impacting on the problem and any solutions.
Risk factor	Something that increases the chance of developing a disease or a condition.
6SQuID	**S**teps in **Qu**ality **I**ntervention **D**evelopment is a framework used to develop interventions in a transparent and systematic way.
Socioeconomic status	A measure of household income, education and occupation.
Sufficient cause	A casual factor with which the effect (outcome) must occur. Often there are multiple components that together become a sufficient cause (sufficient-component causes), as in fire which occurs when there is a combination of heat, oxygen and fuel.
Sustainability	Durability of an intervention which is a direct consequence of the extent to which an intervention is embedded within the systems and routines in which it operates.
System	The set of actors, activities and settings that are directly or indirectly perceived to have influence on or be affected by a given problem situation. Systems include transport, education, health, welfare, housing and families. Many interact with each other.
Theory	A set of statements that organises, predicts and explains observations.
Theory of action	Theory describing how an intervention is constructed to activate underpinning theories of change. See also ACTIVITY/ACTION
Theory of causes	The relationship between causal factors as they exist with system/s and their role in influencing the problem.
Theory of change	Theory describing the mechanisms by which change is expected to occur.
Unintended consequence	An inadvertent positive or negative outcome occurring as a result of an intervention.
Validity	The extent to which the evaluation undertaken and the findings from it are accurate and reflect the truth.
Working theory	Stakeholder understanding of a phenomenon based on local and contextual knowledge and experience.
World cafes	A useful method of co-production to enable group dialogue and decision making. It involves short group conversations to understand the problem in more detail.

INDEX

Page numbers in *italics* refer to Figures and Tables, and those in **bold** relate to glossary entries. Activity or (Activity) in index headings and subheadings may refer to text in Activities or Activity answers.

acceptability, 144–145, **234**
  testing acceptability, 164
action planning, 148, 207
active transport intervention (Activity), 168, *168*
activity (action), **234**
  see also theory of action
adaptation, 49
AIDS, causality, 38–39
  see also HIV infection, causality
alcohol brief interventions (ABI) (as complex intervention), *53*
alcohol consumption, and antisocial behaviour
  causality (Scenario/Activity), 104–106, *105*, 132
  logic model and theory of change, 121–122, *121*, *122*, 123, *124*
  unintended consequences, 125
assets-based approach, 92–94, 142–143, **234**
  overview, *14*, 18–19
  Activity, 143, 153
  to intervention testing, 167–168
  Moving Forward with Gestational Diabetes intervention (case study), 213–214
  Stand Up for Health intervention (case study), 204, *205*
assumptions, in programme theory, 138–141
  Activity, 142, 152–153
  testing assumptions, 163–164

Bedford, M., 180
before and after studies, 42, 187
behaviour (change) theories (scientific theories)
  key theories, 109–116
  levels of explanation and specificity, 117–119
  and problem/causation understanding, 70–71
  theory critique and selection, 117–119

behaviour change wheel, 116, *116*
bias (in intervention evaluation), 188, 189–190, **234**
blinding, 44
Bodkin, A., 19–20
Bradford Hill criteria, 39
Bradley, D., *48*
Bradshaw, J., 61
brainstorming and ranking, 124–125
breakfast choices, causality (Activity), 49, 56–57
Bronfenbrenner, U., 72, 73
Bruton, J. and L., 29

capacity building, and sustainability, 20
cardiovascular disease (CVD), causality, 82–83, *83*
case studies (as evaluation method), *161*
causality and risk factors
  defined, 38, 40, **234**, **237**
  Bradford Hill criteria, 39
  causal loop diagrams, 47, *48*, 77, **234**
  clusters of factors and theory of causes, 92, *92*, **237**
  and context, 50, 69–70, 84, 86–89, *87*, *89*
  distal risk factors, 40–42, 83, 84, 95, **235**
  evidence sources, types and quality, 68–71, 90–91
  factor contributions and prioritisation, 85–91, *87*, 100
  Activity, 90
  and available resources (assets), 92–94
  dangers of over-simplification, 96–98
  ethical concerns, 94–95; *see also* ethics
  political context and influences, 96
  fishbone diagrams *see* fishbone diagrams
  and intervention development (overview), 3–4, 41–42, 54–55

and intervention evaluation (overview), 42–46, *42*
logic models, 74, *76*
modifiable factors *see* modifiable vs non-modifiable and hard to modify factors
multiple causal strands, 50, 51, *52*
necessary causes, 38, **236**
problems as, 71
proximal risk factors, 40–41, 83, 84, **236**
reciprocal/recursive causation, 45, 49, 52, *53*
root-tree diagrams (root cause analysis), 74
single causal pathways, 50
specific problems/interventions
  AIDS, 38–39
  alcohol consumption, *53*
  antisocial behaviour (Scenario/Activity), 104–106, *105*, 132
  breakfast choices (Activity), 49, 56–57
  cardiovascular disease (CVD), 82–83, *83*
  dental caries, *52*
  gender-based violence, 72, *73*
  headaches (Scenario), 36–37, 47
  HIV infection, 40
  hospital admissions following ICU, 74, *75*
  ManaiaSAFE Forestry School (case study), 218–219
  Moving Forward with Gestational Diabetes intervention (case study), 211–213, *212, 213*
  obesity, 40, 41
  school absenteeism, 85–88, *85*, *87*, 91, 92, *92*
  sedentary behaviours (Stand Up for Health) (case study), 98–100, *99*, 126–127, *126*, 202–203, *202–203*
  sleep problems (Scenario/Activity), 80–81, 101–102
  smoking and lung cancer, 38–39
  smoking and young people, 83–84, *83*
sufficient causes, 38, **237**
systems approach and tools, 71–77, *73, 75, 76*
see also theory of causes
champions, 20, 227
change mechanisms
  defined, 108, **234**
  active transport intervention (Activity), *168*
  assumptions, 138–142

coronavirus prevention intervention (care home) (Scenario), *158*
COVID-19 pandemic measures, 136–137, *137*
  Stand Up for Health, *128*, 129, 148–151, *149*
    Activity, 129, 133
  workshop tools, 124–125
  see also theory of change
cluster randomised controlled trials, 185
Cochrane, A., 184
COM-B model, 116, *116*, 121
community gambling, problem analysis (Scenario/Activity), 59–60, 64–66, *64, 65, 66, 78–79*
complex interventions, 3, 52–54, *53*, **234**
  Activity, 54, 57
  development, 54–55, 96–98
complexity and complex systems, 46–49, 52, *53*, **234**
complicated interventions, 51, *52*
  Activity, 54, 58
construct, **234**
contamination of control group, *42*, 44, 185, 186
context
  and causality, 50, 69–70, 84, 86–89, *87, 89*
  historical context, 69–70
  and intervention 'dosage,' 137
  and intervention fidelity, 146–147, 225–226
    Activity, 147, 154–156
  and intervention testing, 168
  and modifiable factors, 84
  political context, 18, 69, 96, 145
    vaccination in India (Scenario/Activity), 70, 79
  stakeholder insights, 86–89, *89*, 140, 141
  and theory of action, 147
    Activity, 147, 154–156
  and working theory, 123
context mapping, 88–89, *89*
contribution analysis, 55
control groups, *42*, 43, 185
  see also cluster randomised controlled trials; randomised controlled trials (RCTs)
convenience sampling, 169–170
co-production and stakeholder engagement
  definition and key features, 23, **234**
  in assumption testing, 140, 141
    Activity, 155–156

challenges, 231–232

for contextual insights, 86–89, *89*, 140, 141

dissemination to stakeholders, 227

engagement techniques and tools *see* workshop tools and engagement techniques

in ethical review, 18

in evaluability assessment, 180

   Activity, 183, *193*

in evaluation, 24

in funding support, *25*, 27, 93

groups and roles (overview), 24–28, *25–26*

   Activity, 31, 34, *34–35*

in identifying effectiveness evidence, 143

in identifying intervention acceptability, 144

importance, 23–24, 232

influence on modifiable factors, 84, 89, 93–94, 142

in intervention testing and adaptation, 167–168, 169, 207

policy makers as stakeholders, *26*, 27

in problem/need identification and understanding, *25–26*, 26–27, 62–67, 69–70, 72, 77

and sustainability, 20, 145, 227

   Activity, 156

team development (process), 28–31, *29*

team norms and cohesiveness, 31

in working theory development, 123–126

see also intervention development team

Corcoran, R., 23

coronavirus prevention intervention (care home) (Scenario), 157–158, *158*, 159, 162, 164, 166–168, 170

   Activities, 162–163, 165, 173

cost-effectiveness and economic evaluations, 176, **234**

COVID-19 pandemic

education and practical guidance, 144

intervention effectiveness, evidence, 143–144

lockdown measures

   ethics, 17–18, 95, 146

   intentions and effectiveness (Activity), 11–12

   legislation, 143–144

   related systems (Activity), 12, 55, 58

proximal and distal risk factors, 41

societal responses, causal loop diagram, 47, *48*

theories and mechanisms of change, 140–141, 147, 154–156

theory of action, 140–141, 147, 154–156

   Activities, 142, 143, 152–153.

unintended consequences of interventions, 146

   Activity, 146, 154

Craig, P., 186, 188

Cross J. E., 29

data protection, 190

Davis, R., 109

dental caries prevention, *52*

determinant, **235**

   see also causality and risk factors

'digital exhaust' data, and evaluation, 181

dissemination *see* reporting and dissemination

distal risk factors, 40–42, 83, 84, 95, **235**

documentary analysis (as evaluation method), *161*

Doi, L., 5

Doll, R., 39

economic evaluations *see* cost-effectiveness and economic evaluations

effect (defined), 184

effect size (significance), 188–189

effectiveness

   defined, 184, **235**

   cost-effectiveness, 176, **234**

   evidence of (from previous interventions), 143–144

   see also intervention evaluation

efficacy, **235**

emergence and emergent properties, 46–47, *53*, 54, **235**

epidemiological evidence, 68–69

ethics, 94–96, 145–146, **235**

   overview, *14*, 17–18

   and intervention evaluation, 178, 189–191

   and intervention testing and adaptation, 167

   see also unintended consequences

evaluability assessment, 176, 179–182, **235**

evaluation *see* intervention evaluation

experimental evaluation designs, 185–186

   see also randomised controlled trials (RCTs); stepped wedge design

experts, as stakeholders, *25*, 27

Facebook, use in stakeholder engagement, 214

factor contributions and prioritisation, **234**

feasibility testing, 159, **235**

    see also intervention testing and adaptation

feedback (loops), 45–46, 47–49, **235**

    causal loop diagrams, 47, *48*, 77, **234**

fidelity

    of intervention *see* intervention fidelity

    theoretical fidelity, 163, 226

    to theory of change, 159, 160, 163, 168, 226

fishbone diagrams, 74, **235**

    hospital admissions following ICU, *75*

    Moving Forward with Gestational Diabetes
        intervention (case study), 211, *212*

    Stand Up for Health (case study), 98–100, *99*,
        126–127, *126*, *203*

focus groups *see* interviews and focus groups

forestry school development (case study),
    216–221

Foster-Fishman, P. G., 46

frameworks for intervention development
    and evaluation

    Intervention Mapping, 5

    MRC Guidance, 5

    PRECEDE-PROCEED, 5, 6

    6SQuID *see* 6SQuID (Six Steps in Quality
        Intervention Development) framework

funders, as stakeholders, *25*, 27

funding issues

    evaluation costs, 21

    stakeholder support, 93

    see also sustainability

gender-based violence, causality, 72, *73*

gestational diabetes and physical activity
    (case study), 210–216, *210, 212, 213, 215*

goal-setting theory, 114, *115*, 129, 151

Grant, R. L., 47, 49

Green, L. W., 61–62

grey literature, 69, **235**

Gubbels, J., 91

Hakimi, S., 19–20

hand hygiene interventions

    and context, 24

    logic model, 108, *108*

        Activity, 122, 132

    and operant learning theory, 111

        Activity, 122, 132

hard to modify risk factors, **236**

Hawe, P., 46

Hawthorne/Observer effect, *42*, 43–44,
    185, 186

headaches, causality (Scenario), 36–37, 47

health belief model, 115, *115*

Health Foundation, 233

health inequalities, **235**

    intervention-generated inequality,
        15–17, *16*

    overview, *14*, 15

Health Inequalities Assessment Toolkit
    (HIAT), 17

Hill, A. B., 39

Hillsdon, M., 97–98

historical context, 69–70

HIV infection, causality, 40

    see also AIDS, causality

HIV treatment and prevention (case study),
    195–201

    causal pathways, logic model, 74, *76*,
        196, *197*

    testing and adaptation, 200–201

    theory of action, 198, *200*

    theory of change, 198, *199*

Hood, R., 47, 49

hospital admissions following ICU, causality,
    74, *75*

Institute of Cultural Affairs, 233

instrumental variable approaches, 186

interrupted time series design, 187, 188

intervention champions, 20, 227

intervention delivery team, as
    stakeholders, *26*, 28

intervention development

    and causality (overview), 3–4, 41–42, 54–55

    and complexity, 54–55, 96–98

    co-production *see* co-production and
        stakeholder engagement

    defining a 'successful' intervention, 14

        Scenario/Activity, 13–14, 34

    frameworks

        overview, 5–6, *6*

        6SQuID framework *see* 6SQuID (Six Steps
            in Quality Intervention Development)
            framework

    future directions, 231–232

    importance, 3–4

nine principles
    overview, 14, *14*
    assets-based approach *see* assets-based
        approach
    ethics *see* ethics
    evaluation planning, *14*, 20–21
    health inequalities *see* health inequalities
    iterative process, *14*, 22–23
    need identification *see* problem/need
        identification and understanding
    sustainability *see* sustainability
    transparent reporting *see* reporting and
        dissemination
    teaching utility of 6SQuID, 228–231, *230*
intervention development team, **236**
    team development, 28–31, *29*
    team norms and cohesiveness, 31
    see also co-production and stakeholder
        engagement
intervention evaluation
    5Ws, 176–179, 182–183, *182*
        Activities, 176, 183, *192*, *193*
    defined, 21, 175–176, **235**
    bias, 188, 189–190, **234**
    blinding, 44
    and causality (overview), 42–46, *42*
    contamination of control group, *42*, 44,
        185, 186
    contribution analysis, 55
    control groups, *42*, 43, 185
    cost-effectiveness, 176, **234**
    data collection methods and methodologies
        overview, 4, 160–161, *161*, 175, 183
        case studies, *161*
        documentary analysis, *161*
        interviews and focus groups *see* interviews
            and focus groups
        natural experiments, 4, 43, 185, 186–187
        non-experimental designs, 187–188
        observation *see* observation (as
            evaluation method)
        quantitative vs qualitative data, 188
        quasi-experimental designs, 186–187
        RCTs, 4, 43, 45, 185–186, 189, **236**
        realist methods, 4
        stepped wedge design, 185–186, 187
        surveys and questionnaires *see* surveys and
            questionnaires

'digital exhaust' data, 181
effect size (significance), 188–189
effectiveness
    defined, 184, **235**
    cost-effectiveness, 176, **234**
    evidence of (from previous interventions),
        143–144
ethics, 178, 189–191
evaluability assessment, 176, 179–182, **235**
evaluation costs, 21
formative evaluation *see* intervention testing
    and adaptation
frameworks
    Intervention Mapping, 5
    MRC Guidance, 5
    PRECEDE-PROCEED, 5, 6
    6SQuID *see* 6SQuID (Six Steps in Quality
        Intervention Development) framework
Hawthorne/Observer effect, *42*, 43–44,
    185, 186
internal vs external evaluators, 182, *182*
Placebo effect, *42*, 43–44, 185, 186
planning during intervention development,
    14, 20–21
purpose and audience, 175–176, 177
    Activity, *176*, *192*
randomisation and matching, 44–45,
    185, 186, 187
reliability, 188
sample size calculation, 189
specific problems/interventions
    ManaiaSAFE Forestry School
        (case study), 220
    traffic calming intervention (Scenario/
        Activities), 174–175, 176, 183,
        192, *193*
and stakeholders, 24, 180; *see also*
    stakeholders: and evaluation
    assessment
    Activity, 183, *193*
and sustainability, 20
testing evaluation elements, 169–172
underlying questions, 183–185, 188–189
and unintended consequences, 177
validity, 188, **237**
intervention fidelity/flexibility, 146–147,
    162–163, 164–165, 225–226
    Activities, 147, 162–163, 165, 173

intervention ladder (Nuffield Council on Bioethics), *16*
Intervention Mapping framework, 5
intervention testing and adaptation
ethics of testing, 167
future evaluation elements (testing of), 169–172
importance and timing, 158–160, 169
intervention fidelity, 161–163
key considerations, 161–167
Activities, 162–163, 165, 173
pilot and feasibility studies, 159
planning testing, 167–168
Activity, 168, 173
process evaluation methods and data, 160, *160*, *161*
testing data collection tools and methods, 170–172
RE-AIM framework, 160, 165–166
specific problems/interventions
coronavirus prevention intervention (care home) (Scenario), 159, 162, 162–163, 164, 165, 166–168, 170, 173
HIV treatment and prevention (case study), 200–201
ManaiaSAFE Forestry School (case study), 220
Stand Up for Health (case study), 207–209, *209*
stakeholder involvement, 167–168, 169, 207
interventions (in general)
defined, 2, 37, **236**
categories of, 50
complex interventions, 3, 52–54, *53*, **234**
Activity, 54, 57
development, 54–55, 96–98
complicated interventions, 51, *52*
Activity, 54, 58
simple interventions, 50, *51*
Activity, 54, 58
see also intervention development; intervention evaluation; *specific problems/interventions; specific types of interventions*
interviews and focus groups, *161*, 178
Activity, 173
testing interview tools and methods, 170–171

IRISS, 233
iterative intervention development, *14*, 22–23

Jepson, R., 5
job interview (theory building), 106–107, *106*

Krueter, M. W., 61–62

Laird, y., 231–232
Leviton, L. C., 4, 179–180, 180–181, 182
literature reviews, 68, 90–91, 117, 139–141, 211
logic models, **236**
overview, 21
for causal pathways, 74, *76*
for outcome chains, 108, *108*
Activity, 122, 132
alcohol consumption and antisocial behaviour, 121, *121*
Stand Up for Health intervention (case study), 127–129, *128*, 148–151, *149*
with theory of action, 148

Maini, R., 107, 121
ManaiaSAFE Forestry School (case study), 216–221
Masquillier, C., 74, *76*, *197*, *199*, *200*
mechanisms of change *see* change mechanisms
meta-analysis, 91, **236**
Michie, S., *116*
mind-mapping, 72, **236**
modifiable vs non-modifiable and hard to modify factors, 82–84, *83*, 85–86, **236**
ManaiaSAFE Forestry School (case study), 219
Moving Forward with Gestational Diabetes intervention (case study), 211–213, *213*
Scenarios/Activities, 81–82, 84–85, 102–103, *102*
Stand Up for Health intervention (case study), 99–100, *99*, 203, *203*
Moving Forward with Gestational Diabetes intervention (case study), 210–216, *210*, *212*, *213*, *215*
MRC Guidance for the Development and Evaluation of Complex Interventions, 5
multi-perspective approach diagrams, 65–66, *66*, **236**
multiple baseline studies, 187

Naidoo, J., 182, *182*
National Institute for Health and Care
    Excellence (NICE), 178
natural experiments, 4, 43, 185, 186–187
necessary causes, 38, **236**
need identification *see* problem/need
    identification
needs assessment, 61–62, **236**
non-experimental evaluation designs, 187–188
nudge theory, 114, *114*
Nuffield Council on Bioethics, intervention
    ladder, *16*

obesity, causality, 40, 41
observation (as evaluation method), *161*
    Activity, 173
Ogilvie, D., 181
operant learning theory, 111, *111*, 119,
    129, 151
    Activity, 122
operationalisation, 137, 148, **236**
    see also theory of action

Parascandola, M., 38
parenting skills intervention, 166
Pennington, A., 23
Petticrew, M., 52–53
physical activity and gestational diabetes (case
    study), 210–216, *210*, *212*, *213*, *215*
pilot studies, 159, **236**
    see also intervention testing and adaptation
Placebo effect, *42*, 43–44, 185, 186
policy makers, as stakeholders, *26*, 27
political context, 18, 69, 96, 145
    vaccination in India (Scenario/Activity),
        70, 79
population, target *see* target population
PRECEDE-PROCEED model, 5, 6
preventive interventions (defined), 50
problem/need identification and
    understanding
    overview, *14*, 15, 60
    community gambling (Scenario/Activity),
        59–60, 64–66, *64*, *65*, *66*, *78–79*
    needs assessment, 61–62, **236**
    pre-identified problems, 60–61
    problems as risk factors or outcomes, 71
    stakeholder involvement, *25–26*, *26–27*,
        62–67, 69–70, 72, 77

and sustainability, 20
systems approach and tools, 71–77,
    73, *75*, *76*
workshop tools, 63–67, *64*, *65*, *66*, 77
process evaluation methods and data, 160,
    160, *161*
    testing data collection tools and methods,
        170–172
    see also intervention testing and adaptation
programme theory (defined), 107, **236**
    see also logic models; theory of action;
        theory of change; theory(ies)
propensity score matching, 45, **236**
proximal risk factors, 40–41, 83, 84, **236**

quasi-experimental evaluation designs,
    186–187
questionnaires *see* surveys and questionnaires

randomisation and matching, 44–45, 185,
    186, 187
randomised controlled trials (RCTs), 4, 43, 45,
    185–186, 189, **236**
reach of intervention, testing, 165–166
RE-AIM framework, 160, 165–166
realist evaluation methods, 4
reciprocal/recursive causation, 45, 49, 52, *53*
recruitment (testing), 169–170
regression discontinuity approach, 186
reliability, 188, **237**
remedial interventions (defined), 50
reporting and dissemination, *14*, 21–22,
    227–228, **235**
    dissemination methods, *228*
    planning for impact, 233
    TIDieR-PHP reporting guidelines,
        22, 138, 227
research study designs, 68–69, 90–91
    see also randomised controlled trials (RCTs)
resources available *see* assets-based approach
rich pictures, 63–65, *64*, *65*, 89, **237**
risk factors *see* causality and risk factors
Rod, M. H., 55
Rogers, P. J., 50, 52
root-tree diagrams (root cause analysis), 74

sample size calculation, 189
sampling strategies, 169–170
Sanson-Fisher, R. W., 183, 188

school absenteeism, causality, 85–88, *85, 87,*
   91, 92, *92*
school meals interventions, 20
sedentary behaviours *see* Stand Up for Health
   intervention (case study)
self-efficacy theory of motivation, 112, *112*
significance, in intervention evaluation,
   188–189
simple interventions, 50, *51*
   Activity, 54, 58
6SQuID (Six Steps in Quality Intervention
   Development) framework, **237**
   overview, 5, 6, *6*
   applying to day-to-day problems, 224
   applying to existing interventions, 224–225
   compared with other frameworks, 5–6
   Steps 1 & 2 (problem and causes)
      see causality and risk factors; modifiable
      vs non-modifiable and hard to modify
      factors; problem/need identification and
      understanding
   Step 3 (change mechanism and theory) *see*
      change mechanisms; theory of change
   Step 4 (theory of action) *see* theory of action
   Step 5 (testing) *see* intervention testing and
      adaptation
   Step 6 (evaluation) *see* intervention
      evaluation
   use in teaching, 5, 228–231, *230*
   whole process (case studies)
      HIV treatment and prevention, 195–201,
         197, 199, 200
      ManaiaSAFE Forestry School, 216–221
      physical activity and gestational diabetes,
         210–216, *210, 212, 213, 215*
      real-world lessons, 201, 209, 216, 221
      Stand Up for Health, 201–209, *202, 203,*
         205, 206, 208, 209
Skinner, E. A., 109
sleep problems, causality (Scenario/Activity),
   80–81, 101–102
smoking and lung cancer, causality, 38–39
smoking and young people, causality,
   83–84, *83*
smoking cessation interventions
   and causation, 38, 84
   defining 'success' (Scenario/Activity),
      13–14, 34
   ethics, 18, 95

Sniehotta, F. F., 41
social desirability bias, 190
social norms theory, 114, *114,*
   121–122, *122*
social-cognitive theory, 113, *113*
socio-ecological model of health, 72, *73,*
   109–110, *110,* 119
   and causal pathways, 72, *73*
socioeconomic status, 15, **237**
   see also health inequalities
spot/acne prevention intervention
   (fictional example), 42, *42*
stakeholder engagement *see* co-production and
   stakeholder engagement
Stand Up for Health intervention (case study),
   201–209
   Activity, 129, 133
   factor identification, 98–100, *99,* 126–127,
      126, 202–203, *202–203*
   resource assessment, 204, *205*
   and sustainability, 121
   testing and adaptation, 207–209, *209*
   theory of action, 151, 204–207, *208*
   theory of change logic model, 127–129, *128,*
      148–151, *149,* 204, *206*
stepped wedge design, 185–186, 187
sufficient causes, 38, **237**
sugar tax, and complex systems, 47, 49
surveys and questionnaires, *161*
   accessibility issues, 178, 190
   bias and (im)partiality, 189–190
   pre-existing questionnaires, 171, 190
   testing and development, 171–172
sustainability, **237**
   overview, *14,* 19–20
   and co-production, 20, 145, 227
      Activity, 156
   and ongoing refinement, 226–227
   and theory of action, 145
   and theory of change, 119–121,
      120, 145
systematic reviews, 68, 91, 211
   see also literature reviews
systems and systems approach
   defined, 46, **237**
   complex systems, 46–49, 52, *53,* **234**
   importance and overview, *14,* 20
   mapping tools, 63–65, *64, 65,* 71–77,
      73, 74, 75

specific problems/interventions
  COVID-19 pandemic measures (Activities),
    12, 55, 58
  school meals interventions, 20
  traffic calming interventions,
    20 per cent rule
  stakeholders in, *26*, 28
  systems dynamic approach, 77

target population
  recruitment and sampling (testing),
    169–170
  as stakeholders, *25*, 26–27
  testing intervention reach and engagement,
    165–166
team development (process), 28–31, *29*
team norms and cohesiveness, 31
testing and adaptation *see* intervention testing
  and adaptation
theoretical fidelity, 163, 226
theory of action, **237**
  action planning, 148, 207
  and context, 147
    Activity, 147, 154–156
  'dosage,' 135, 137
  key considerations, 138–146
  operationalisation, 137, 148, **236**
  specific problems/interventions
    active transport intervention
      (Activity), *168*
    coronavirus prevention intervention
      (care home) (Scenario), 158, *158*
    COVID-19 pandemic measures, 140–141,
      142, 143, 152–153., 147, 154–156
    HIV treatment and prevention (case
      study), 198, *200*
    ManaiaSAFE Forestry School (case study),
      219–220
    Moving Forward with Gestational Diabetes
      intervention (case study), 214, *215*
    Stand Up for Health (case study), 151,
      204–207, *208*
  and sustainability, 145
  vs theory of change, 107, 135–136, 147
  utility of TIDieR-PHP framework, 138
  workshop activities and tools, 204–207
    Activity, 156
theory of causes, 92, *92*, **237**

theory of change, **237**
  behaviour (change) theories
    (scientific theories)
    key theories, 109–116
    levels of explanation and specificity,
      117–119
    and problem/causation understanding,
      70–71
    theory critique and selection, 117–119
  change mechanisms *see* change mechanisms
  COVID-19 pandemic measures, 136–137, *137*
  fidelity to, 159, 160, 163, 168, 226
  specific problems/interventions
    alcohol consumption and antisocial
      behaviour, *124*
    coronavirus prevention intervention
      (care home) (Scenario), 157–158, *158*
    HIV treatment and prevention
      (case study), 198, *199*
    Moving Forward with Gestational Diabetes
      intervention (case study), 214
    Stand Up for Health (case study), 127–129,
      128, 148–151, *149*, 204, *206*
    Well!Bingo, *120*
  and sustainability, 119–121, *120*, 145
  vs theory of action, 107, 135–136, 147
  and unintended consequences, 125–126
  working theory, 123, 123–126, **237**
  workshop tools and engagement techniques,
    124–125, 214
theory of planned behaviour (TPB), 110–111,
  110, 117, 118
theory(ies) (in general)
  defined, 106, **237**
  see also specific theories; specific types of theory
TIDieR-PHP reporting guidelines, 22,
  138, 227
traffic calming interventions
  evaluation (Scenario/Activities), 174–175,
    176, 183, *192*, *193*
  systems approach, 20
transtheoretical model of change, 112, *113*
Tuckman, B., 28

unintended consequences, 125–126, 127,
  146, **237**
  Activity, 146, 154
  and intervention evaluation, 177

and intervention testing and adaptation,
        166–167
see also ethics
United Nations Evaluation Group (UNEG),
        175, 177

vaccination
    as a complex intervention, 53
    ethics, 94–95
    political context (Scenario/Activity), 70, 79
    as a simple intervention, *51*
validity (in intervention evaluation), 188, **237**
Veinot, T. C., 16

Waterlander, W. E., 77
Weed, D. L., 38
Well!Bingo intervention, 119, *120*
Wholey, J. S., 179–180
Wight, D., 5, 72, *73*, 217
Wilkie, M., 217, 218
Wills, J., 182, *182*
Wimbush, E., 5
working theory, 123, 123–126, **237**

workshop tools and engagement
        techniques
    Activities, 90, 103, 155–156
    brainstorming and ranking, 124–125
    context mapping, 88–89, *89*
    Facebook, 214
    fishbone diagram development, 74
    mind-mapping, 72, **236**
    multi-perspective approach diagrams, 65–66,
        66, **236**
    rich pictures, 63–65, *64*, *65*, 89, **237**
    root-tree diagram development, 74
    world cafes, 66, **237**
        case study, 67
    see also co-production and stakeholder
        engagement
world cafes, 66, **237**
    case study, 67
World Health Organisation and United Nations
        Evaluation Group (UNEG), 21

youth unemployment intervention (Activity),
        31, 34, *34–35*